Coping with Radiation Therapy

Coping with Radiation Therapy

A Ray of Hope

Daniel Cukier, M.D.
AND
Virginia E. McCullough

Lowell House
Los Angeles

Contemporary Books
Chicago

Library of Congress Cataloging-in-Publication Data
Cukier, Daniel.
    Coping with radiation therapy: a ray of hope / Daniel Cukier and
Virginia E. McCullough.
       p. cm.
    Includes bibliographical references and index.
    ISBN 1-56565-147-2
    1. Cancer—Radiotherapy—Popular works. I. McCullough, Virginia.
II.Title.
RC271.R3C85   1993
616.99'40642—dc20   92-34430
                                           CIP

Requests for such permissions should be addressed to:

    Lowell House
    2029 Century Park East, Suite 3290
    Los Angeles, CA 90067
    Publisher: Jack Artenstein
    General Manager: Bud Sperry
    Director of Publishing Services: Mary D. Aarons
    Text Design: Tanya Maiboroda

Manufactured in the United States of America

10 9 8 7 6 5 4 3 2 1

Contents

Dedication

TO PAST patients who inspired me to write this book; to current patients who encouraged me to see the project through; to future patients whose travails will help me to continue growing professionally and as a human being.

And to my wife, Joan, in gratitude for her usual love and support.

Acknowledgments

THERE ARE numerous people who helped make this book a reality. First and foremost, I'd like to thank my coauthor, Virginia McCullough, whose professional expertise and wisdom brought the text to life over the years it took to think and rethink it and make it right. Lu Buckmaster's computer skills were so valuable to us as we went through all those revisions and her dedication and tireless efforts will not be forgotten. Lyle Steele and Jim Kepler recognized the need for this book early on and found it a home, and Janice Gallagher and Lynette Padwa were helpful and insightful editors. I also want to thank all the folks at the New Jersey Chapter of the American Cancer Society, particularly John King and Maureen Alex, for their encouragement and assistance. Julia Schopick's personal and professional wisdom has also been valuable in our efforts to bring the book to the attention of patients who need it. My appreciation also goes to my typists, who never failed to meet my deadlines: Bonnie Dairomondo, Audrey Shaw, Eileen Del Vecchio, and Kathy Spillane.

Finally, mention is due to the manufacturers of the therapy machines. Their high standards of quality and the dedication of their sales and service staff are invaluable to the radiation therapist. Special thanks to the people at Siemens, Varian, and General Electric.

—Daniel Cukier, M.D.

A Word to Professionals

THE goal of this book is to help cancer patients and their families and loved ones understand the process of radiation therapy. I believe that patients are better able to cope with their illness and recommended medical treatment when they are given comprehensive information about both. Therefore, I've written the book in a style that lay people can easily understand. Where the use of medical terminology is unavoidable, I've made every attempt to explain the concepts in a way that the average reader can grasp. The brief discussions of chemotherapy and surgery are approached in the same way.

It is my hope that the many professionals who work with cancer patients and their families will discuss in greater detail the issues raised here. While radiation therapists quite naturally attend to the emotional concerns of their patients, many other practitioners do so as well. Clinical social workers often establish a close therapeutic relationship with patients and their families. Hospital oncology nurses and home-care nurses frequently advise patients and help them cope with the physical and emotional side effects of radiation treatment. Dietitians may be involved in planning nutritional programs for patients.

No matter which profession we practice, we all want not only to provide quality care to our patients, but to help alleviate their fear and anxiety as well. Offering concise, easy-to-comprehend information about the treatment they are undergoing is one way we can achieve this.

The radiation dose schedules and treatment times vary somewhat among different treatment centers. Much depends on the patient's clinical picture. Thus, the doses and times described in this book are only general guidelines, so that the patient is given an approximate idea of what to expect.

—Daniel Cukier, M.D.

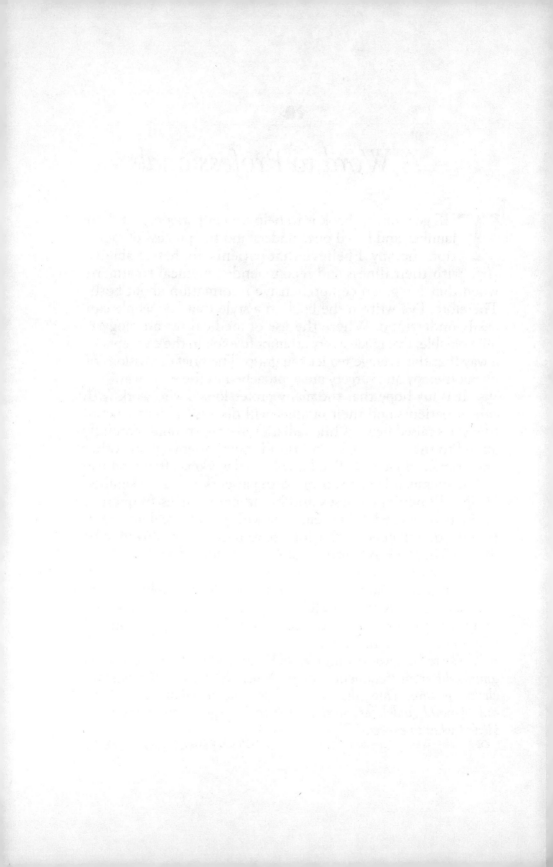

Introduction

MORE THAN likely, if you are reading this book you either have cancer yourself or are close to someone who does. You may have already been referred to a facility for radiation treatment, following a series of diagnostic tests and consultations with your physicians. The past few days or weeks have been traumatic, and now you're about to begin radiation treatment—a treatment about which you surely have dozens of questions. And you may be lonely and frightened as you prepare to cope with the treatment you will be undergoing in the coming weeks.

This book was written to provide cancer patients and their loved ones with the information they need to cope with radiation treatment. (Only those cancers most commonly treated with radiation are discussed. Similarly, pediatric cancer is a specialized field and is not included because of those unique issues.) My goal is to make the course of your treatment a little easier by providing you with basic knowledge. You'll know why and, just as important, *how* the treatment is done. You'll know what to expect at the time of treatment, and you'll be prepared for the most commonly experienced side effects and have effective ways to alleviate them.

Your own physician has probably told you what to expect, but after you left his or her office, you may have thought of many more questions. You may also still be going through the natural adjustment period when you learn to accept your illness and the treatment plan that has been recommended for you.

Since radiation therapy usually begins as soon as possible after cancer is diagnosed, you may have little time to prepare psychologically for treatment. This book will explore the normal emotional ups and downs you may experience during the course of your treatment. It will also offer advice about sorting through your feelings about your illness and its effect on your body, as well as its impact on your relationships with family and friends. The information in this book will serve a twofold purpose. It will fill the gaps in the information you have, and it will help you form the questions you want to ask your own physicians.

Naturally, the ability to cope with cancer and radiation therapy varies greatly from person to person. Having the support of family members and other loved ones is crucial during this period. No disease puts stress on a family quite like cancer does, and family relationships are often stretched to the limit. Some families grow closer; others are torn apart. Helping the patient and family members is an essential element of the radiation therapist's job.

Your radiation therapist will usually be involved in your case from three to six weeks, so he or she won't be providing ongoing support over long periods of time. However, radiation therapists are not simply involved in the technology of your treatment. They can also help patients cope with side effects, adjustments in lifestyle, nutrition, and so on.

I've been a radiation therapist for over 30 years and have learned that a well-informed patient recovers more easily than one who is kept in the dark. Furthermore, many remarkable recoveries occur every day, even among patients whose cancer is in an advanced stage. So while statistics may be important when discussing overall outlook with a patient, I always emphasize that an individual's response to treatment determines the final outcome.

RADIATION THERAPY AND ITS SIDE EFFECTS

In order for you to understand how radiation treatment works, the first chapter of this book will explain why radiation treatment is performed and take you step by step through treatment planning. While the treatment itself is painless, the equipment may look forbidding, and you may be afraid of the *idea* of radiation being directed to your body. This chapter will help alleviate your fears and answer questions you may have about treatment procedures.

The side effects of radiation therapy are predictable and, most important, they are almost always manageable. You will be less fearful after you have read chapter 2 and learned what symptoms you can expect to experience and at approximately what point during treatment they are likely to appear. Most side effects occur in the general area of the body receiving the radiation. For example, radiation directed to the prostate may cause urinary tract symptoms because of the proximity of the urinary bladder to the prostate gland. While some symptoms are unavoidable, changes in diet, specific medications, and some adjustments in lifestyle can alleviate them.

THE GROWING ROLE OF SUPPORT THERAPIES

The conventional therapies for cancer—surgery, chemotherapy, and radiation—are considered primary treatments. In a technical sense, these treatments are external to the patient. That is, they are done *to* a person and *for* a person. However, nowadays we know that patients can do much on their own behalf. Maintaining a positive psychological outlook and using mental imaging to boost the immune system can be powerful tools of recovery. Diet can also make a patient more comfortable during treatment and enhance the effectiveness of the therapy. These are generally considered "support" therapies, used in conjunction with conventional cancer treatments.

The crucial role of a patient's mental outlook has taken on special importance in recent years. It is common knowledge among physicians and lay people that a cancer patient who is basically cheerful and optimistic will do better than a patient with a negative and pessimistic personality. We now have scientific evidence to show that a positive outlook creates subtle biological changes that can boost the immune system and allow the body to fight off the invading cancer. In other words, while the will to live has always been respected *subjectively*, we are beginning to accumulate *objective* evidence to prove how important it is for cancer patients. In recent years, a technique known as guided imaging or visualization is used to help patients gain a sense of control over their illness. The fear of the unknown may also be reduced, which in itself fosters a positive attitude. Meditation and biofeedback techniques are also useful.

While support therapies are extremely helpful, I don't believe that cancer patients should rely only on special diets and mental imaging techniques to cure their disease. There is simply no body of evidence to support the contention that these methods are effective *when used alone*. However, much is still unknown about the body's ability to fight the disease of cancer. We do know that any technique that boosts the immune system can only help, it can never hurt. Therefore, I stress the importance of these treatments when used along with conventional therapies.

LIVING WITH CANCER

A patient's illness isn't an isolated event, and part of your radiation therapist's role is to advise you about your day-to-day life during treatment. Chapter 3 is devoted to a discussion of lifestyle issues, with a special emphasis on diet. The food you eat may have a considerable effect on your body's ability to fight cancer. Certain foods may make some side effects worse; other foods may help alleviate symptoms. This chapter offers suggestions about cooking, food selection, and so on. Physical activity, sexual interaction, sleep and rest habits, and social relationships all affect your well-being, and these issues are also discussed.

EMOTIONAL CONCERNS

Two patients with the same disease in the same stage may have totally different reactions and side effects, depending on their perception of their conditions. Their ability to function during the course of radiation treatment can be profoundly affected by the presence or absence of anxiety. Fear about the future, questions about the possibility of recovery, financial concerns, and special pressures on relationships with others are all issues with which cancer patients must contend. For some patients, support groups are the answer; other patients choose individual psychotherapy to help them cope; still others rely on spiritual counselors and family or friends for support. Chapter 4 will discuss the profound emotional issues that invariably accompany a diagnosis of cancer.

RADIATION TREATMENT FOR SPECIFIC CANCERS

Radiation treatment plans vary greatly, depending on the kind of cancer being treated, other treatments being used, and individual factors such as age and overall physical condition. Treatment times and doses also vary among treatment centers and according to the patient's clinical picture. Chapter 5 is designed to help you learn about radiation treatment for your specific cancer. An entire section is devoted to each type of cancer for which radiation therapy is commonly recommended. In addition, I discuss specific expected side effects and their treatments. Diet and lifestyle issues and some emotional concerns that often accompany particular cancers are also discussed in each section. However, I urge you to read the introductory chapters that provide more general information before turning to the individual sections.

I believe that it is important for physicians to be as positive as possible when discussing treatment and the possibility of cure. Therefore, without being unrealistically cheerful, I attempt to describe the origin and stage of a patient's cancer as concretely as possible, knowing that when a patient is able to get a clear understanding of their disease, the fear of the unknown is often greatly reduced. This in turn lays the groundwork for a patient to gain a feeling of control over the condition and not simply be a helpless observer. To that end, I've included as much information as possible to help you understand the origin and course of your particular cancer.

The statistics concerning the incidence of certain cancers, the effectiveness of treatments, and cure rates for various cancers change often. Therefore, for most of the cancers mentioned in this book, it is nearly impossible to provide meaningful cure or long-term survival statistics—what is valid today might not be valid tomorrow. The outlook for your particular case should be discussed with your own physician.

WHEN CANCER HAS SPREAD

Of course, cancer may metastasize, or spread beyond its original site, and when this occurs, radiation therapy is generally used to control the disease, rather than cure it. This is known as palliative treatment, and it is primarily used to control pain or to prevent damage to organs, such as the liver and brain. Chapter 6 describes the specifics of treatment delivered to the parts of the body most likely to be treated for metastatic cancer. In addition, I also discuss side effects and relevant diet and lifestyle issues.

CHEMOTHERAPY

Chemotherapy—the treatment of cancer with chemical agents —is often given before or following a course of radiation therapy. In certain cases it is given in conjunction with radiation therapy. In chapter 7, I've listed some common chemotherapeutic agents currently used to treat cancer, along with the expected side effects and possible complications.

No other area of cancer treatment is changing more rapidly than chemotherapy. In addition, some substances are used to help the body's own defense systems fight the disease, while others may actually help make radiation treatments more effective. The reverse is also true, and radiation treatment may enhance the ability of chemotherapy to cure or control some cancers.

HANDLING PAIN

Chapter 8 discusses pain, the most dreaded symptom of cancer. Radiation treatment can alleviate much of the pain caused by certain cancers, and it is often given for this purpose. However, many cancer patients may also need medications. About 95 percent of patients should have their pain well controlled with radiation and medications. Cancer specialists know how to use medications judiciously and can prescribe them individually or in combination, thereby minimizing their side effects.

Because you are part of the treatment team, you should play a role in deciding which medication you prefer and, in effect, take charge of your own problem with pain. This book will answer your questions about pain-relieving medications and their side effects. I will also talk about possible addiction to these drugs, a concern of many patients.

Nowadays, there is simply no reason to suffer discomfort and pain in silence. If one drug or combination of medications isn't effective, others are available to try. Unrelieved pain can make treatment more difficult because of physical stress, and it may also affect the way in which patients are able to cope with their illness. Therefore, it is important for you to know that the pain you experience can and should be relieved.

DIAGNOSTIC TESTING

A variety of tests are used to diagnose cancer, monitor progress of the treatments used, and to follow up after treatment is completed. It is likely that during the coming years you will be undergoing, on a regular basis, various x-ray tests and the newer diagnostic tests using non-x-ray technology. I've included a thorough description of these tests in chapter 9 so that you will understand why they are ordered and the procedure used to perform them.

YOUR RIGHT TO KNOW

It's unfortunate but true that many patients and family members are afraid to ask questions. Perhaps they fear hearing an answer that will be psychologically threatening, or they are afraid to ask questions that might make them appear stupid. But when it comes to radiation therapy, there is no such thing as a stupid question.

I'm often asked such questions as "Will radiation make my hair fall out?" or "Will I become radioactive because of the radiation therapy?" A wife might ask if she is at risk of getting cancer by having sexual relations with her husband, who is undergoing treatment for prostate cancer. Some people have an underlying fear that the radiation will kill them, usually because they know about the extensive fatalities at Hiroshima and Nagasaki. Are these stupid questions? Not at all. They are valid questions that deserve answers. In my experience, patients have questions about everything from hair loss to sleep disturbance to sexuality. Therefore, I've included a chapter at the end of the book that answers many of the most frequently asked questions about radiation therapy and cancer.

Patients also want to know if radiation treatment is a last-ditch effort or if they have good chances of recovery. They are concerned about being bedridden and incapacitated, and they may wonder if some other treatment could have been used instead of radiation. Family members may be frightened by the patient's loss of appetite or signs of depression. Each of these issues is discussed in appropriate chapters which, when taken together, will help patients and their families cope throughout an entire course of radiation treatment.

THE PATIENT IS IN CHARGE

In my view, it is absolutely essential that all cancer patients understand the disease process taking place. They must believe they are part of the treatment team, and they must demand to be fully supported in the effort to restore their health and make them as comfortable as possible during treatment.

As a patient you are entitled to the standard of care that this book presents. It *is* available. If you are dissatisfied with your radiation treatment center, speak to your referring physician. He or she will locate another radiation therapy facility for you. Keep in mind that ultimately you choose your physicians and support services, and that it is up to you to take an active part in decisions affecting your recovery.

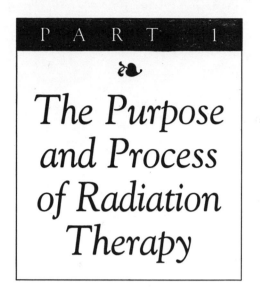

PART 1

*The Purpose
and Process
of Radiation
Therapy*

Chapter 1

The Basics
of
Radiation
Therapy

THE USE of radiation for diagnostic and treatment purposes was a revolutionary step in the evolution of medicine. Without it, we wouldn't be able to diagnose numerous conditions and diseases, and we wouldn't be able to treat cancer with radiation. Diagnostic x-rays allow us to view the inside of the body without invading it—literally bringing the inside out. Therapeutic radiation takes the technology one step further and allows us to treat cancer in various organs without opening up the body. For some kinds of cancer, radiation is the predominant form of treatment. For other types, it is used in conjunction with surgery and/or chemotherapy.

Because we are able to detect some cancers earlier than we used to, an aggressive combined treatment approach aimed at curing the cancer often has been found to be more effective than using only one or another treatment. For example, early detection of breast cancer by means of mammography has for many women meant less drastic surgery along with radiation to treat the breast. Chemotherapy may also be administered to decrease the possibility of distant spread.

The rapid advances in radiation and computer technology have resulted in improvements in treatment accuracy and results. At the same time, there are fewer and less severe side effects than experienced even a few years ago.

How Does Cancer Develop?

Cancers begin as a cluster of cells multiplying in an out-of-control manner, unlike the body's normal cycle of cell destruction and replenishment. Particular abnormal genes (oncogenes) that influence this uncontrolled growth have been identified in some cancer cells.

Scientists believe that once a cluster of cancer cells has arisen in an organ, there is a step-by-step progressive pattern in cancer growth and spread. At first, the body's immune system resists the growth of the invader, a process that may take years. Once the battle tips in favor of the cancer, local growth proceeds. At some point, and this point is thought to vary among cancers as well as individuals, the cancer spreads locally into 8surrounding tissues. The next step is for cancer cells to attach themselves to and penetrate the neighboring blood-vessel and lymph-vessel walls.

Once the cancer cells have penetrated the blood-vessel wall, they enter the bloodstream and the lymph system of the body. Cells traveling in the lymph system settle in the lymph nodes. The cancer cells then travel throughout the body, but must reattach to and penetrate the vessel wall at a distant site. The organs into which these cells settle are generally those richly endowed with blood vessels and with nutrient materials. Thus, the bones, the liver, the lungs, and the brain are common sites for metastases.

How Does Radiation Treatment Work?

The effects of radiation on tissues and their cells are very complex. For the sake of simplicity, the principles can be explained as the ability of radiation to injure the genetic material (DNA) in the center (nucleus) of the cell. The results of the biochemical effects, which *do not* make the body radioactive, is to either destroy the cell or alter its metabolism so as to hinder its ability to function normally.

Radiation may be administered in the form of gamma rays or x-rays (as discussed later). They differ only in their origin, but not in their ultimate biological effects.

Radiation therapy is administered to those cancers where there is a selective ability for the radiation to destroy cancer cells while allowing the adjacent normal cells to repair themselves from the injury.

The reason that the treatment course for some cancers is so relatively long is to allow for normal tissue repair and to minimize permanent injury. *Relatively* small doses given over a long period of time allow for normal tissues to recover at the expense of the cancer cell. (Tissue repair can also be helped by proper nutrition and patients' mental state. These issues will be discussed in this book.) The daily dose must also be great enough to destroy the cancer cell while "sparing" the normal tissues. This "balancing act" forms the basis of modern radiation therapy, which has been further complicated in recent years because, in many cases, chemotherapy, which also harms normal tissues, is used in combination with radiation.

Patients often ask why some cancers can be destroyed by radiation while others don't respond to this treatment. Simply stated, cancer cells vary in their *sensitivity* to destruction by x-rays. This sensitivity largely depends on the *origin* of the cancer. For example, a skin cancer is generally more sensitive, meaning more easily destroyed, than a cancer originating in the brain.

The sensitivity may also vary in the same cancer *site*. One patient with cancer of the uterus may respond much better to radiation than another patient with the same cancer because the uterus contains more than one cell type. Each cell type varies in its ability to be destroyed by radiation therapy. Thus, cancer cells arising from the lining of the uterine cavity are more sensitive to radiation than those arising from its muscle cells. As a result, a relatively small amount of radiation may be necessary to effectively treat one patient, whereas much higher doses are necessary for another.

In addition, cancer cells in the same tumor may vary in their sensitivity to radiation depending on their *location* in the mass. Generally the outer areas of the tumor are more sensitive.

This is related to the amount of oxygen reaching the cancer. The peripheral regions are better oxygenated and are destroyed more easily than tumor cells at the center.

When we talk about *resistance* we mean the opposite of sensitivity. Some cancers, such as melanoma, a type of skin cancer, are usually resistant to radiation therapy and little or no benefit is achieved by using it.

Treatment Planning

The decision to use radiation therapy for your cancer was arrived at after consultations between the pathologist, surgeon, internist, and chemotherapist, all of whom are part of your treatment team.

Some cancers respond better to surgical treatment or chemotherapy (treatment using drugs or other chemical agents). Nowadays, improvement in cancer survival often involves treatments that combine surgery, radiation, and chemotherapy. But each situation is individualized—or tailored—to the particular patient. In addition to the type and location of the cancer, your age and general physical condition guide the choice of treatment procedures used.

Organs are composed of different cell types—each type can lead to a different cancer. For example, cancer cells arising from the air sacs of the lungs lead to a different type of cancer than those arising from the bronchial tubes. The cell type provides the information that allows a radiation therapist to predict the tumor's response to radiation. Thus, a prognosis, or educated opinion, about the probable effectiveness of radiation therapy is determined.

The individual cell type may vary in its ability to spread. This degree of aggressiveness is referred to as cell *grade*.

We also look at the extent to which the cancer is present. Is it *localized*, meaning limited to the organ of origin, or has it spread to neighboring or distant sites in the body? The evaluation of the extent of the cancer is referred to as the *staging* of the tumor. This involves using various diagnostic x-ray tests (see chapter 9). CT scans and nuclear scans, ultrasound examinations, and simple x-ray tests are often used to assess the entire situation. Obviously, the goal is to correctly treat the tumor while minimizing any negative effects on the surrounding normal tissues.

We use the three parameters of grade, type, and staging to evaluate how much radiation will be necessary and for what period of time. This is known as the *dose-time* relationship of treatment. The *dose* levels and length of treatment are guidelines. The treatment schedules have been arrived at by the cumulative experience of major treatment centers, using large numbers of patients. *However, every person's case is individualized, and your treatment dose and time may vary from those described here.*

Your radiation therapist won't treat your cancer as an isolated event. He or she generally works closely with the referring physician before and during your treatment, jointly evaluating the impact of the therapy on your entire medical condition. For example, other diseases and disorders may coexist with cancer, or you may have medical problems that could be aggravated by radiation therapy. These conditions must be carefully monitored.

In addition to delivering treatment, your radiation therapist is also responsible for treating the side effects of the treatments with appropriate medications. Your nutritional status is monitored, and you will be given advice about certain food groups that should be avoided and those you should emphasize (see chapter 3). In other words, your radiation therapist is involved with your overall well-being during and after radiation therapy.

Consulting with Your Radiation Therapist

A radiation therapist is a physician, specifically a radiologist, who is specially trained in not only the science, but the art, of administering radiation treatments. Some radiologists are certified in both diagnostic and therapeutic radiology. With the current emphasis on subspecialization, most radiologists are either diagnostic or therapeutic radiologists. A radiation therapist is trained to evaluate which patients may undergo radiation therapy by determining if the tumor will respond to radiation.

When you and your family members first meet with your radiation therapist, tell him or her what you already know about your illness. I generally ask patients, "What do you understand about your disease?" I also tell them that by the time they leave my office they should have a complete understanding of their cancer and its treatment. You should leave the radiation therapist's office with the knowledge that you are part of the treatment team.

Write your questions down before your office visit, because the issues you want to discuss might slip your mind when you're actually in the office. This is understandable because the first visit is often emotionally charged for both you and your family members. If you think of additional questions when you are back home, call the physician and get your answers. All this information will alleviate your fear, lower anxiety, and therefore boost the therapeutic effect of radiation.

Don't be afraid to ask the radiation therapist or your other physicians about the likely outcome of your disease. Such issues should be dealt with realistically. Your radiation therapist's response should be based on current *statistics* for the specific cancer and its stage. However, it's just as important to discuss individual variation. I often mention cures that I've seen in my own practice even when, according to the statistics, the outlook was grim. As Norman Cousins wrote in his book *Head First*, "Don't deny the diagnosis, just the verdict that is supposed to go with it."

No preparation is necessary before going to the radiation therapist's office. It's important, however, to have as many records available as possible. These include previous history and medical examinations related to the cancer and other conditions as well as any available X rays and other tests. If you can't personally obtain these, then make sure they have been sent to your radiation therapist's office beforehand. This will save a lot of time.

During the initial consultation, the radiation therapist will review the pathology report and all x-ray tests available, and evaluate and determine an appropriate field (portal) of treatment. This is drawn on your skin with indelible ink. This ink may wash off with time, and you will be instructed not to scrub at the marks but to shower or bathe normally. A simulator machine will ensure that the portal will include the cancer and its potential areas of spread.

This phase of treatment planning is known as *simulation*. Thus, the treatment process is set up, checked, and rechecked to guarantee that the *actual* treatment will be as precise as possible. In addition, any questions about the treatment plan can be resolved with you and your treatment team, including the technical staff, who are an important part of delivering radiation therapy.

As you discuss your condition with your physicians, bear in mind that treatment plans for cancer can't be isolated from a person's age, general physical condition, or even his or her psychological makeup. An older person who is suffering from cancer in addition to having an underlying chronic health problem—a lung condition, for example—will be treated differently than a person 20 years younger with a similar cancer but without other physical disabilities. Although there's no universally accepted definition of quality of life, it certainly enters into decisions about radiation dose levels, length of treatment, and size of treatment areas.

Your radiation therapist will probably be involved in your case for an average of two to eight weeks. The time to build a comfortable relationship with this person is at the beginning of treatment.

Treatment Procedure

Radiation treatments do not involve pain or any other sensation. Although patients are afraid they will feel intense heat, there is no heat, light, or sound associated with the treatment. (The fact that treatment is "silent" may produce anxieties of its own.) However, the information in this book will help alleviate any anxieties you may have.

The patient lies on a treatment couch for a few minutes. The exact length of time depends on body size, the location of the tumor, and the size of the area being treated. The area subject to the treatment is known as the *treatment field*.

The treatment equipment unit you see is mostly shield and/or circuitry. When the machine is turned on, the beam is of a predetermined size to pass through to the desired site.

You are able to breathe normally during treatment. This is surprising to some patients, but ordinary breathing does not significantly alter the position of the organs. Physical restraints are generally not used unless a patient is disoriented and unaware of his or her surroundings and therefore lacks normal judgment. Young children, senile older persons, and severely ill patients may require some immobilization devices or tranquilizers.

Today's treatment rooms look pleasant and cheerful. Some patients wish to have music piped in the room during the few minutes of treatment to break the silence. If you wish, ask your radiation therapist if this can be done for you. In general, every effort is made to keep you comfortable and relaxed. Patients are usually relieved after the first treatment because they see how painless and easy the actual treatments are.

If you're too ill to travel on your own, then arrange for friends, relatives, or an ambulance service to take you to the radiation therapy facility. Naturally, if you're an inpatient, you will go to the facility by direct in-hospital transportation.

You may wonder whether you can drive back home after the first treatment or subsequent treatments. You may also be concerned about feeling very sick after the first treatment. Except where there is a physical disability to preclude driving, there is no need to make unusual arrangements. (However, those people having radiation therapy to the brain are advised not to drive because, by virtue of the cancer itself, these patients are at risk for a sudden turn for the worse.) Unless you have been told not to, you can drive yourself home after the first treatment and usually after subsequent treatments.

Portals, or areas of treatment, vary in size depending on the staging of the tumor and a person's body size and shape. A heavier person will require a longer daily treatment time than will a small person because of the greater amount of tissue present between the skin surface and the tumor. However, the treatment course is the same. Treatment times average just a few minutes, depending upon the dose necessary. Two to four minutes is standard, although it may be even shorter.

Treatments are usually administered through both the front and the back of the body, or as a single treatment through front, back, or side. Alternatively, multiple-angle treatments are sometimes necessary, as well as rotation of the machine around the body. Some patients require a combination of these different treatment approaches. This depends on the particular clinical situation and is determined by your radiation therapist.

Treatments are, as a rule, given five consecutive days each week, and the entire treatment course lasts several weeks. On average, the treatment course time will vary from two to eight weeks. You will receive a total dose of radiation, which is then referred to in terms of daily dose. The concept of daily doses is medically known as *fractionation*.

The neck, chest, abdomen, and pelvis (soft tissues) generally can't tolerate more than 900 to 1,000 units per week, 180 to 200 units per day. The bones of the arms and legs can easily tolerate daily doses of 250 to 300 units. (Radiation units are technically called Grays or Centigrays.) More rapid treatment may lead to severe short- or long-term side effects. Conversely, lower doses or a longer course may result in decreased effectiveness of radiation therapy. Thus, there is an optimal dose and time schedule for treating various types of tumors.

The length of treatment courses and the radiation doses have been established through extensive clinical trials. Modification of this time-dose may be necessary if problems arise because of complications with the cancer itself, the side effects of radiation, or a person's general physical condition.

Following an initial consultation, a letter is mailed to the doctors on your treatment team to summarize your condition, describe the treatment plan and expected side effects, and make recommendations for further tests if indicated. Periodic letters and telephone calls follow during the treatment course when indicated. Depending on their condition, patients are usually examined by the radiation therapist many times a week.

After your radiation therapy is completed, a discharge letter is mailed to your various doctors describing the side effects;

possible problems; progress; and recommendations. Many radiation therapists, I among them, see patients for one or more
follow-up visits after treatment is completed. Remaining problems and side effects can be addressed, and patients have an
opportunity to ask additional questions. In my experience,
patients feel less abandoned and are able to easily make the
transition from radiation treatment to general medical care
when they know that a connection to the radiation therapist
can continue.

You have a right to feel both physically attended to and
emotionally supported during the course of your treatment. The
technicians working with you, as well as the radiation therapist,
should be available to answer questions and help you with the
"mechanics" of treatment. If, at any time, you believe that you're
not being given the kind of information and help you need, then
by all means speak up!

This advice applies to family members, too. If a loved one is
undergoing radiation treatment, you may be better equipped to
ask questions and retain information than the patient. In addition, if you will be caring for your family member, much sound
advice can be directed to you. Confusion about diet, sleep patterns, activity levels, treatment of side effects, and so on can be
avoided when all who are involved with the patient are aware of
medical advice and suggestions. Furthermore, your own fears
may be alleviated by taking an active role in your loved one's
treatment.

Equipment and Dosage

Most common x-ray *tests* are performed with x-ray energies mea-
sured in thousands of volts. Radiation *treatments*, by comparison,
usually involve energies of over one million electron volts.

In the past 25 years, new machines have been designed to
increase the power, or energy, of the x-ray beams. Prior to the
early 1960s, x-ray treatment units had powers of approximately
200,000 volts. These earlier x-ray therapy treatments were
accompanied by many untoward side effects. One of the worst
was skin damage.

The new so-called super voltage therapy units fall into two main categories. The first, Cobalt 60, is an isotope. It is a radioactive substance emitting approximately one million electron volts of energy in the form of gamma rays. The second is the Linear accelerator machines, which deliver an energy range of 6 million to 18 million volts of x-rays.

In the interest of clarity and to keep these explanations as simple as possible, the Cobalt 60 and Linear accelerator units can be considered as one entity, both being super voltage machines. This is appropriate because their ultimate therapeutic properties are similar. And for the sake of simplicity, I refer to the dosages of radiation as units. However, these are technically known as Grays (Gy). For example, 10 Grays (Gy) equal 1000 Centigrays (CGy).

Super voltage units have some definite characteristics important to treatment. For one, they are "skin sparing," meaning that little radiation affects the skin surface. Most of the x-ray energy goes to the tumor. However, the tissues in the path of the x-ray beam are also irradiated.

Secondly, with the modern equipment, there is minimal *scatter* of x-ray energy outside the treatment beam. By scatter, we mean the presence of radiation in the body outside the field of treatment. If you picture a beam of light from a powerful flashlight projected on a wall, the visible beam of the light is well defined (equivalent to the radiation beam) with only a slight halo of light around the edges (equivalent to the scatter). In radiation therapy, a sharply defined x-ray beam minimizes the side effects of treatment because only small amounts of radiation travel to other parts of the body.

With Linear accelerator machines, the sharpness of the beam edge allows for very precise treatment, and adjacent tissues are spared unnecessary radiation during treatment. The precision a radiologist can achieve with these machines is similar to that necessary in surgical procedures. Lastly, the Linear accelerator may be programmed to treat with electrons rather than x-rays for special situations, which are described later.

The Support Staff

Radiation therapy is delivered with the assistance of a team of specialists who assist the radiation therapist. *Radiation physicists* accurately determine the radiation doses and precisely assess the risk of injury to normal tissues. Radiation physicists are experts in medical computer technology, and with today's complex treatments, this expertise is essential in treatment planning.

Radiation technologists operate the complex treatment machines, position the patient for treatment, and verify that treatments are precisely reproduced daily. They combine their technical and scientific skill with compassionate "hands on" involvement with the patient.

Oncology nurses are nurses whose specialty is working with cancer patients. They have received extensive training in order to deal with the multitude of concerns patients have, including such things as fears about treatment, controlling side effects, changing dressings, intravenous feedings, and so on.

These three disciplines are an integral part of today's radiation treatment, and you should feel free to ask questions about the role they will play in your care.

Modern Treatment

At one time, radiation therapy caused more severe side effects than it does today. Much technological progress has been made over the past decades, and now advances in radiation therapy have contributed to improvement in the cure rates for many cancers. Still, your apprehension is normal and expected, and you should not be satisfied until *all* your concerns are addressed and your questions answered. Your radiation therapist is there to help you during your treatment course, and I urge you to ask about all aspects of the treatment you are receiving.

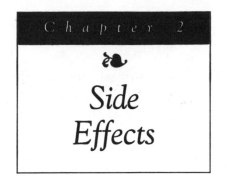

Side Effects

I'M OFTEN ASKED, "If radiation treatment is so sophis-ticated today, why are there still side effects?" It's true that medical science has made enormous strides in improving the delivery of radiation, and the area of the body being treated with radiation is far more precisely targeted than ever before. However, some facts about radiation haven't changed.

Although the radiation beam travels directly to the target area to be treated, it also affects organ tissues in its path. For example, if someone's uterus is being treated, the x-ray beams will need to pass through the large intestine, the small intestine, and bladder to get to the uterus. There is simply no way to move the tissues internally to allow one organ to receive the radiation exclusively.

It is the tissue that is in the way, so to speak, that reacts to the irritating effects of radiation. The next logical question is, "Are the normal tissues being affected by radiation going to be permanently damaged?" The answer to this question goes back to the reason radiation therapy is so often successful.

There is a fundamental difference in the way tumor cells and normal cells react to radiation. In those patients whose can-cers are considered treatable with radiation, tumor cells are much more sensitive to radiation than are the surrounding nor-mal cells. Thus, the side effects are caused by the generally reversible damage to the normal surrounding cells. This is true whether the cells are located on the same organ being treated or on other tissues in front or in back of the tumor.

So, in essence, when we talk about radiation sickness or radiation side effects, as they are now called, we mean the effect of the radiation beam on tissues surrounding the organ affected by cancer. Most patients experience side effects for only a short time, generally restricted to the course of radiation treatment. These are called *acute* side effects. They should disappear within two to three weeks following the completion of radiation treatment. However, particularly when there are underlying pre- or coexisting conditions, especially involving the intestines or the urinary bladder, the symptoms may never completely go away and then they are called *chronic* side effects. Fortunately, only a small number of patients experience long-term side effects, which can range from mildly annoying to severe.

Side effects vary, of course, depending on the part of the body to which the radiation is targeted. This chapter provides an *overview* of the side effects a patient might experience, but a more detailed discussion will be found in later chapters, which discuss treatment of specific kinds of cancer. This overview will give you enough background to make the chapters in Part 2 beneficial. Remedies to combat the side effects mentioned here will also be discussed in greater detail in later chapters. Therefore, don't be alarmed if you don't completely understand the particular symptoms described here or the ways to alleviate them. Simply refer to the appropriate chapters in this book for more information.

There is great variation among individuals in severity of side effects. For example, one person may experience severe diarrhea or cramping with a particular dose of radiation, while another person receiving the same dose reports only mild symptoms. I've had numerous patients tell me that the lack of side effects caused them to question whether the radiation treatments were working. However, there is no relationship between the severity of the side effects and the effectiveness of the treatment. Some people are simply more fortunate than others, and their bodies are able to tolerate the radiation treatments without causing significant discomfort.

The following sections describe typical side effects of radiation treatment, beginning with the brain and continuing to the rest of the body.

TREATMENT TO THE HEAD AND CHEST

When radiation is administered to the *brain*, there is often a temporary swelling of brain tissue, because of water retention. The water retention enlarges the brain tissue just enough to expand slightly against the rigid bones making up the skull. A cortisone-type medication will usually alleviate this swelling, so most patients do not report any symptoms. A few people, however, may begin to experience severe headache, visual changes, or projectile vomiting. When this occurs, the medication is immediately increased and the radiation dose is modified.

Many patients will complain of sleepiness and a sense of being a bit confused or disoriented for an hour or two after radiation treatment to the brain. A short nap is usually beneficial, and the disorientation disappears shortly after waking. The next day, treatment can continue without difficulty.

When radiation is administered to the brain for longer than three or four weeks, most people will begin to notice hair loss. If a small area is being treated, hair loss is confined to that spot. If the entire brain is being treated, hair loss occurs over the whole head. However, there is individual difference in the strength of hair roots, and the degree of loss varies from one person to another. Length of the treatment course and the dose will also affect the probability of hair regrowth.

Radiation to the *face and neck* usually results in the gradual thickening of saliva within two to three weeks after treatment begins. The amount of saliva is frequently reduced as well, and the patient's sense of taste is often diminished and altered.

Tumors in the face and neck usually require high doses of radiation for about five to seven weeks. Therefore, the salivary changes are progressive. Patients often complain of having a very dry mouth, difficult and painful swallowing, and a general loss of appetite. Artificial salivary products are now available and usually help, and liquid diets are often a good way to get needed nutrition and avoid the irritation of eating solids. Drinking fluids frequently and sucking on lemon drops—or a similar kind of hard, sour candy—often helps.

Anesthetic gels are available to soothe membranes in the mouth and throat if they become irritated. This side effect is often accompanied by loss of appetite and therefore, inadequate nutrition, and it is crucial that the symptom be treated. Because the skin may redden somewhat, cortisone creams and skin balms are generally helpful. We also recommend using sun block during the summer months to protect the skin from ultraviolet rays, which accentuate the effects of radiation on the skin.

Radiation to the *chest* area will also cause some swelling in the esophagus—the tube through which food passes when we swallow. The radiation irritates this area, and a patient may experience it as heartburn or a lump in the throat or chest. This can be controlled by avoiding extremes in temperature of food and liquids and ingesting only lukewarm beverages and food. Chewing food extremely well so that it can travel through the esophagus easily is also helpful. Patients are generally told to avoid alcohol and spicy foods, both of which can irritate the esophagus. Judicious use of liquid antacids also helps this condition.

Increased coughing and mucus production in the chest and throat result from irritation to the trachea and bronchi. Both home and medical remedies are available to alleviate these symptoms. Skin creams are also used on the skin of the chest if mild reddening occurs.

TREATMENT TO THE UPPER ABDOMEN

Patients experience nausea and indigestion when receiving radiation to the *upper abdomen* (above the navel). These symptoms begin one to two weeks into treatment, and cause loss of appetite, so it is important to treat them. The nausea can be controlled with various medications, some of which are similar to preparations used for motion sickness. Indigestion can be treated with both medication and diet. If not controlled, these symptoms lead to loss of appetite. Since a patient's nutrition is important to recovery, these concerns must be addressed. Food choices and amounts are discussed in chapter 3.

TREATMENT TO THE LOWER ABDOMEN (BELOW THE NAVEL)

When we administer radiation to the pelvic area, the small and large bowels are always in the path of the targeted organ. This is the case regardless of the angle of the beam, which is why most patients will begin to experience diarrhea by the second or third week of treatment. Because radiation to organs in the lower body usually requires five to six weeks of treatment, controlling the diarrhea becomes important for maintaining good nutritional status and comfort. Fortunately, we do have a variety of medications available to try. (All are discussed in subsequent chapters.)

Radiation to the *rectal* area often results in additional side effects, irritation to the anal opening being one. Cortisone creams that relieve this symptom are available. Sometimes the rectum will spasm, and this is usually relieved by cortisone suppositories.

The *bladder* will often undergo spasm because of radiation. A patient will feel the need to urinate frequently even when there is almost no urine in the bladder. Thus, even a small amount of urine in the bladder creates a need to empty the bladder, and the patient experiences what is known as urinary urgency and frequency. Medications are available to alleviate these symptoms and make the patient more comfortable.

HOW RADIATION AFFECTS YOUR SKIN

Many years ago, radiation therapy often caused significant damage to the skin. Sometimes the skin would ulcerate and a scar was formed when it healed. (Occasionally these open sores didn't heal.) The radiation equipment used today delivers x-ray energies that don't cause major damage to the skin.

Some people, particularly those who are fair skinned, may see some reddening of the skin, especially when higher doses are used. The skin on the neck, for example, will often become inflamed. A small raw area may be produced, particularly in places where the skin rubs together—under the arms, in the folds between the thighs, the buttocks, and beneath the breasts.

Creams that contain lanolin will soften and moisturize the skin. (Nivea cream works well.) If a small area of skin actually peels and looks raw, a one-percent cortisone cream is effective. It reduces irritation while it promotes healing. When the skin becomes itchy, the old standby home remedy of cornstarch seems to work best. It can be used in a bath or applied topically with a towel or a bandage.

There are many remedies for skin irritation—don't think you must live with it. Ask your physicians to recommend products that they know have worked well for their patients.

FATIGUE

One nearly universal side effect of radiation treatment is an overall feeling of fatigue or malaise. Exactly when this fatigue begins and how severe it becomes varies from patient to patient. However, it's *not* connected with the severity of the disease. The fatigue is probably caused by the passage of cellular debris out the body; this debris is the product of the breakdown of the tumor and normal tissues that results from the radiation treatment. I stress the fact that this fatigue is not related to the activity of the disease, but to the radiation treatment itself.

Nevertheless, when patients begin to feel tired, they invariably believe they are getting worse, not better. Even optimistic and cheerful people will experience this and begin to worry. However, in the vast majority of cases, this fatigue is a side effect of the radiation and not a sign or symptom of worsening disease. Furthermore, it promptly reverses itself within two to three weeks following completion of radiation therapy.

CHANGES IN BONE-MARROW CELLS

Another side effect that must be carefully monitored involves changes in the bone-marrow cells. These cells reproduce very rapidly and are also extremely sensitive to radiation, and the treatment may depress the marrow's ability to function normally. As a result, the white and red blood cells and platelets, which are formed in the marrow, may not be released into the bloodstream in adequate amounts.

The CBC (complete blood count) will determine if the red and white blood cells and platelets are lower than normal. In some cases, we need to temporarily discontinue radiation treatment in order to allow the blood count to return to a normal range. Because radiation treatment is often used in combination with chemotherapy, it becomes even more important to watch for this abnormality.

No specific symptoms usually accompany a low white blood-cell count, but the patient may be more susceptible to infection. A lowered red blood-cell count may cause dizziness and fatigue. (Again, the symptoms of fatigue must be evaluated to see if it is the normal fatigue accompanying radiation treatment.) Very low platelet counts will cause areas of hemorrhage, usually first noted on the skin, appearing as blotchy bruised spots.

Not all bone-marrow elements are necessarily affected in the same way. Some patients may show lowered white cell counts, but the red cell count remains normal. The reverse can also occur. The white blood count is the most sensitive index by which to judge bone-marrow activity. When you wonder why you are having still more blood drawn, it is likely that your blood counts are being monitored so that bone-marrow activity can be assessed.

REPRODUCTIVE AND SEXUAL ISSUES

Women and men in reproductive years must pay special attention to certain side effects unique to this age group. Women who undergo radiation treatment to the pelvic region will lose ovarian function two to three weeks into treatment. In essence, they have an artificial menopause, which may be permanent. A surgical procedure called oophoropexy, which moves the ovaries out of the way of the radiation beam, is often performed if maintaining fertility is an important issue. Fertility is of special concern for young women who have cancer of the reproductive organs or Hodgkin's disease. (See individual sections in chapter 5.) Surgery, chemotherapy, and radiation therapy may affect fertility, temporarily or permanently. Therefore, all patients for whom future childbearing is an issue require fertility counseling prior to beginning treatment.

Young men must also deal with fertility concerns, particularly those with testicular cancer, Hodgkin's disease, and non-Hodgkin's lymphoma. In some cases, sterility occurs as a result of these diseases, for reasons not well understood. In addition, chemotherapy may cause sterility that cannot be reversed. Radiation to the pelvic area, even when not aimed at the testicles, will result in some radiation "scatter" reaching them. Scatter is the radiation energy that is transmitted outside the field of treatment. So, even when the testicles are not directly treated, decreased sperm production and motility may lead to sterility. In addition, there is the potential for genetic damage, which could result in birth defects in future offspring. In these situations, storing sperm in a sperm bank prior to the onset of radiation treatment is a reasonable solution if a family is desired in the future.

Sexual functioning is an important issue for cancer patients. Women with cervical or uterine cancer may experience sexual difficulties because radiation treatments have resulted in scarring of the vaginal tissues. Men with prostate cancer may become impotent as the result of surgery (although less frequently than in the past) or radiation. (See chapter 5.) Because these side effects are limited to particular cancers, I have included more detailed information in the appropriate sections.

Potential fertility and sexual dysfunction are issues that should be thoroughly discussed before you begin treatment. In many cases, you will have options and the time to explore them before making treatment decisions.

LONG-TERM SIDE EFFECTS

Obviously the goal of radiation treatment is to control or cure cancer existing in a particular site. Both the *daily* dose of radiation and the *total* dose have an impact on the ultimate outcome. Over the past decades, guidelines have been established for maximizing the benefits while attempting to minimize the long-term effects of radiation on the body's tissues and organs.

Long-term side effects of *abdominal* radiation are injuries to the small intestine, including narrowing, ulceration, and abnormal connections between small bowel loops (*fistulae*). The resulting symptoms may not show up for several months to many years after radiation treatment, but when they occur, surgery may be required. Fortunately, the incidence is fairly low—approximately 5 percent of all patients undergoing radiation treatment to the abdominal area. The large intestine may be similarly affected.

A slightly larger group of patients, about 10 percent, (particularly patients with bladder or prostate cancer) will eventually have some *bladder* damage when that organ has received radiation. These patients experience urgency and frequency of urination because the bladder does not distend appropriately. No satisfactory cures are currently available. More rarely, a patient will experience some bleeding in the bladder, which may require cauterization.

Some scarring of the lung during radiation treatment to the *breast and chest* may result in persistent respiratory symptoms. The breast tissue may also scar and result in changes in the way the breast feels when touched. Recent reports have suggested that radiation treatment delivered to the chest for Hodgkin's lymphoma may cause an increase in the incidence of breast cancer, particularly among younger women. Radiation delivered to this part of the body may, depending on the dosage, result in damage to the heart and its blood vessels.

Treatment to the *head and neck* may leave saliva production deficient and taste sensations altered. In addition, persistent tooth decay and gum and bone infections may be long-term problems. While rare, some patients experience a decreased range of motion in opening and closing the mouth, which is a result of damage to the temporomandibular joint.

At one time, scarring of the skin tissues was a more common long-term side effect of radiation. However, this is becoming less frequent because of the advances in radiation technology.

One particular long-term complication of radiation that is not currently well understood is *immunosuppression*. What this means is that radiation may significantly alter the body's ability to defend itself against infection and subsequent cancers. This is usually seen when treatment areas are large. For example, patients who have been cured of lymph-gland cancers (lymphomas) may, many years later, be more susceptible to the onset of new cancers.

At this point in cancer treatment, we are continually trying to balance the potential for cure with the risks of treatment. It isn't always easy to do, especially in this era when we sometimes combine radiation and chemotherapy with the hope of enhancing the potential for a complete cure. Yet, we must be cautious, because we want to minimize the possibility of long-term side effects.

Chapter 3

Diet and Lifestyle During Therapy

THE DISEASE of cancer and its treatments often alter patients' ability to meet nutritional needs and to continue their normal lifestyles. Therefore, administering radiation treatments, or any other cancer therapy, requires that we work with patients in order to help them feel as well as possible during treatment and to take advantage of the body's own natural mechanisms to fight the disease.

The information presented below is directed to family members as well as to patients. Furthermore, it is important that those who are involved in the day-to-day care of a cancer patient understand the reasons why modifying the diet is so important.

APPETITE AND RADIATION THERAPY

The physical and emotional stress created by cancer treatments lowers the body's natural defenses. In addition, the cancer cells compete with the normal cells for survival, further lowering these defenses. The body's ability to handle this stress is known as immunocompetence.

Proper nutrition will enable your body to better handle the stress brought on by surgery, chemotherapy, or radiation. In practical terms, a good diet helps you feel better throughout the treatment. There is no question that adequate intake of vitamins

25

and minerals, particularly zinc, has an effect on the immune system's response to cancer. Laboratory research with animals has demonstrated this, and much experimental work is currently being done on humans to establish the importance of nutrition in cancer therapy. (See the reading list on page 200 for additional information.)

Loss of appetite is a symptom of cancer itself, although we are not sure why. We do know that there is a central regulatory system for hunger and satiety. (The exact way this system is activated in the brain is still unknown.) It is known that cancer produces chemicals and alters metabolic functions, so as to interfere with the body's system for regulating appetite. This creates a vicious cycle. The patient has little appetite, but nutrition is essential to help combat the cancer and the effects of treatment.

As discussed in the previous chapter, the common side effects of radiation (particularly for that given to the abdomen and pelvis) are nausea, diarrhea, and loss of appetite. Furthermore, some patients undergoing radiation therapy (or any cancer treatment, for that matter) become anxious and depressed, which can also cause their appetite to diminish. As you can see, loss of appetite is a constant risk for a number of reasons. Cancer patients must be diligent about getting the proper nourishment.

The degree to which you'll experience loss of appetite depends on which area of your body is being treated, the size of the treatment field, and the overall treatment dose. For example, a patient receiving radiation to the mouth will often experience drying of the mouth and loss of taste, but will not be nauseated. Patients receiving radiation to the chest may complain of discomfort when the food passes through the esophagus. A patient whose abdominal region is receiving radiation will complain more about nausea than loss of taste or dry mouth. When radiation is given in the pelvic area, diarrhea, cramping, and bladder symptoms are more troublesome than nausea. These symptoms result in diminished appetite.

Most people are able to continue eating food by mouth during radiation therapy. Otherwise intravenous feeding, called hyperalimentation, is required. High-calorie solutions are administered through a tube inserted in a vein. This form of feeding may be needed for a period of several weeks, during which the patient is hospitalized. The patient is carefully monitored for signs of blood clots or infection that can result from irritation to the vein.

ADJUSTING TO DIETARY CHANGES

Altering the diet is an essential part of the overall treatment plan for a patient undergoing radiation therapy. For example, commercially available artificial saliva to combat dryness in the mouth allows food to be swallowed and pass through the esophagus more smoothly. While the food may still taste bland, the act of eating will become less of a chore, and the patient will feel better physically and emotionally.

It's crucial that cancer patients and their families adjust to new eating patterns. This usually means breaking away from the adage that three square meals are best. In fact, a patient undergoing radiation therapy is much better off eating "like a bird." Birds eat small amounts of food all through their waking hours and get exactly what they need. My patients feel much better if they don't schedule regular meals, but instead eat when they feel like it. Six to eight small meals a day, or some variation on constant nibbling, seems to work best.

Sometimes well-intentioned family members and friends urge their loved one to eat. In fact, they may literally try to force food on the person, only causing further worry and strain. The whole subject of nutrition for a cancer patient must be treated rationally, because emotions tend to get in the way and family members overreact.

The "food is love" connection is often so strong that I've seen patients literally berated for not accepting the copious amount of food being prepared. Family members may feel quite helpless, and fixing elaborate meals is the one tangible thing they can do to help the person's physical recovery. But exhortations such as "You have to eat to get your strength back" are rarely compelling to a person who has no appetite.

Mike Simmons, a 22-year-old man with Hodgkin's disease, a cancer of the lymph nodes, was receiving radiation treatments to the chest and abdomen. By his third week of treatment he was still somewhat nauseated in spite of the medication he was taking to counteract it. Mike's mother had already seen him lose considerable weight as a result of his disease, and she was understandably concerned when he didn't care to eat.

Mrs. Simmons thought the best thing she could do for her son was to fill the kitchen with his favorite food—steak and potatoes, pancakes, and hearty sandwiches. She was distressed and disappointed when her son simply refused to eat these foods.

Mike developed symptoms common to many cancer patients. First of all, he developed an aversion to meat. It is well documented that cancer patients often experience a change in their taste buds that causes them to find meat proteins unappealing. Secondly, the aroma of food triggered nausea. Food aromas, particularly when trapped in steam beneath cooking pots and chafing dishes, can be particularly troublesome. Even before the patient has touched a morsel of food, the aroma alone can cause nausea. Mike was also upset when faced with large amounts of food.

For many cancer patients, the idea of sitting at the table three times a day is nothing less than an "assignment." They begin to become anxious when large amounts of food are placed in front of them, and this is made worse when the food aromas are mixed. Mike was able to gain some weight when he began using a blender to make many cold drinks. I encouraged him to make these drinks whenever he felt like it, not on any exact time schedule. These drinks consisted of many nutritious substances such as vegetables, fruits, and juices. Shakes made from low-fat ice cream are a good source of calories for those who can tolerate dairy products. Mike also ate cold soups and nibbled on small amounts of cold cooked vegetables and fruit. When he felt better, he gradually added foods until he was again eating normally.

Many patients will feel like eating a small plate of food, supplemented with liquid drinks. Nearly all pharmacies carry commercial liquid nutritional preparations (Sustical, Ensure,

Carnation, Vivonex) designed for patients who, for whatever reason, have difficulty with solid food.

One of my patients, a 75-year-old woman with cancer of the esophagus, had become disgusted with a liquid diet. I advised her to try eating commercially available pureed baby foods instead. They are tasty and provide adequate nutrition. This patient eventually put on some weight and was able to improve the quality of her life. Patients can also mash their own home-cooked foods. If their sense of taste has been altered or diminished they may wish to season food more heavily than usual.

For the most part, people receiving radiation therapy feel better if they eat vegetable rather than animal protein. Excellent sources of vegetable protein include cooked dried beans and legumes, peas, corn, and soy products. Most natural food stores and many supermarkets carry a product called textured vegetable protein, which is spun soybean fiber. Generally, this soy product is mixed with other foods and is considered a substitute for animal protein.

Some cancer patients do tolerate fish protein as well as poultry, as long as the skin (fat) is removed. Again, each individual serving need not be large. Many small amounts throughout the day are best.

Pasta, rice, and potatoes are excellent sources of calories, although fatty or spicy sauces should be avoided. Some pasta is fortified with protein, making it even more valuable in the diet.

Fresh vegetables should be cooked rather than eaten raw. Raw foods tend to create too much bulk in the diet and aggravate the irritation of the small and large bowels already created by the radiation therapy.

I also urge patients not to use beverages containing caffeine (an intestinal stimulant)—coffee, tea, hot chocolate, soft drinks, and so on. Herbal teas and decaffeinated coffee, tea, and soft drinks (regular or diet) should be substituted.

Most radiation therapy patients can use alcohol in moderation, one drink of wine or beer a day. Exceptions include those with a preexisting problem with alcohol or other medical reasons (i.e., acute bladder, prostate, and throat problems) it should be avoided. Beer provides extra calories, and a glass of wine in the evening may actually relax a person for restful sleep.

I recommend that you take multiple vitamin and mineral supplements, particularly the group of nutrients known as the B-complex vitamins, and vitamins C and E. These vitamins assist the body's own defenses in fighting the cancer and the stress of radiation and other therapies. Liquid vitamin supplements are available for patients receiving treatment to the neck or chest, which may make swallowing capsules difficult.

SOME SPECIAL CONSIDERATIONS

During radiation therapy some patients experience nausea and occasional vomiting, but this side effect is usually not severe and can be easily controlled with medications. The nausea usually begins after the first or second week of treatment. When you alter your diet, the dosage of antinausea medication can often be decreased. But it generally isn't effective to simply treat the nausea and then expect the patient to eat normally, meaning three full meals a day. A combination of dietary changes and medication works best. In some cases, antinausea medication can be taken in suppository form.

Diarrhea can also be a problem for some patients. To control it, I recommend limiting the amount of fat in the diet. We've found over the years that fat is poorly absorbed by patients and delays the emptying of the stomach. Therefore, many frozen dinners and packaged foods should be eliminated from the diet because they tend to be high in fat content.

Radiation therapy may also cause some gastrointestinal enzyme (lactase) deficiencies resulting in intolerance to lactose, the sugar in milk. When lactose is no longer properly digested, water is attracted to the intestine, ultimately causing intestinal irritability that results in watery diarrhea.

Under normal conditions, the cells in the intestinal tract lining slough off very rapidly. Radiation therapy only aggravates this process. The turnover of the cell lining may be so great that small ulcers occur and an inflammation of the intestine, called enteritis, takes place. This condition also leads to lactose intolerance, which means that some patients can't ingest milk and other dairy products without risk of irritation and diarrhea. Because lactose is used as a sweetener in many prepared foods and as a filler in many drugs, it's important to become a careful label reader.

Lactose intolerance varies so much from individual to individual that trial and error is the only way to tell if dairy products can be comfortably eaten.

DIET AND MEDICATION WORK TOGETHER

Diet and medication work together to relieve the side effects of radiation therapy. It's possible to reduce your need for medication with a proper diet. On the other hand, to refuse the safe medications we now have available and to try to control side effects with diet alone generally isn't satisfactory. Be sure to discuss your diet with your radiation therapist who is familiar with the specific details of your case.

Most important, don't allow food to become a source of anxiety or conflict. Those involved with the patient's care should *not* take control of the person's diet, particularly the amount of food eaten or the timing of the meals.

The reading list in the back of this book provides sources of information about dietary adjustments and cancer. You can also ask to be referred to a hospital dietitian who has experience advising cancer patients and their families about these issues.

LIFESTYLE CHANGES

We can loosely define *lifestyle* as the kinds of activities a person undergoing radiation therapy will feel like doing, balanced by the amount of rest he or she will need. As mentioned earlier, patients receiving radiation therapy will often experience an overall sense of fatigue. Neither patients nor those around them should become alarmed. Although we aren't sure why this dragged-out feeling occurs, we know that it isn't related to the severity of the cancer. It does not mean that the disease is getting worse.

GETTING THE REST YOU NEED

Naturally, getting adequate rest is a priority during radiation therapy. When fatigue appears a week or two into treatment, I generally advise listening to what your body tells you, and resting. This does not mean actually sleeping. When possible, it is better to move about during the day, perhaps even taking a walk if it isn't inadvisable for other medical reasons. For some patients, a *short* daytime nap is beneficial.

You will probably notice that sleep doesn't relieve the kind of fatigue the radiation therapy induced. (The exception is, of course, when the brain is being treated. In that case, sleepiness is natural and a nap is usually refreshing.) If you give in to the fatigue and sleep during the day, you may have trouble sleeping at night. This sleep pattern will then make you out of step with the rest of the family and the outside world. It sets up a situation that causes strain on your family and friends, who want to be available to help out. However, if they are carrying on their normal activities during the day and trying to stay up with an ill person during the night, it can prove to be too much for them.

The night hours are often dreaded by cancer patients—after all, we are all more vulnerable to our emotions at night. If a person is already anxious and somewhat depressed, these feelings will be amplified when the house is quiet and others are sleeping. Suffering from physical symptoms combined with the fear of pain can turn the night into a very bleak time. A patient's problems become a loved one's problems too, and the next day might be even more difficult.

When a person has trouble falling asleep or staying asleep, altering the time of the evening doses of medication can help. I recommend taking the medication approximately an hour before going to bed for the night. You will get the maximum benefit from the medication, allowing you to fall asleep while you are comfortable. This is true if the medication is for pain, nausea, diarrhea, or bladder irritation. The goal should always be to have a restful night.

Home remedies that are recommended for people suffering from insomnia are worth trying. These include a warm bath before retiring, a glass of wine, a cup of herbal tea or a glass of warm milk (if milk is tolerated well), listening to a relaxation tape or soothing music, and so on.

It is very important that sleep disturbances be dealt with, because studies have shown that sleep disorders are detrimental to the body's ability to fight disease and infection. Sleeping pills are sometimes useful, and they are best prescribed by your family doctor, who is familiar with your overall physical condition. If you have any questions about sleep problems, by all means discuss them with your primary-care physician.

PHYSICAL ACTIVITIES

By using a combination of diet and medication, most patients undergoing radiation therapy should be able to remain alert during the day and enjoy mild physical activity. However, as with diet, well-intentioned relatives and friends may actually try to push the ill person too far. Patients are the best judges of just how much activity they can tolerate. There is nothing to be gained from "working through" the disease with excessive exercise.

Walking is probably the best overall exercise, and I encourage my patients to walk as much as they believe they can. Again, you, as the recovering person, are the best judge. Walking also gets you out of the house and into the fresh air. In addition, the exercise may stimulate the appetite, and increased food intake can lead to greater feelings of well-being.

Many employed persons continue working, usually keeping up with their normal schedules. I've found that most people want to work if they can because it keeps them out in the world and allows less time to dwell on the illness or feel sorry for themselves. Maintaining a normal lifestyle also provides a boost in self-esteem and overall mental attitude, which in turn may strengthen the immune system.

Patients are able to work because most side effects of radiation treatment are *not* debilitating, although they may be annoying and require medication and adjustments in diet. Of course, if the disease itself is severe, patients may need to alter their work schedules.

I believe it is crucial for cancer patients to participate in social activities as much as possible. The disease itself may make them feel severely isolated, and cutting off all regular interaction with friends and family only makes this feeling worse. For some people, the interaction with people in self-help and support groups (discussed in the next chapter) may be integrated into a normal, if somewhat modified, lifestyle. Moreover, those who have always been religious should stay in touch not only with friends from their church or synagogue, but with their spiritual counselor. This is the time to call on all one's support systems.

Hobbies and creative activities, such as art and music, may bring pleasure and joy. Studies have shown that these kinds of activities may stimulate areas of the brain to secrete chemicals beneficial to the healing process. Basically, the goal is for you to feel as much a part of normal life as possible. While it's pointless to deny the fatigue, depression, pain, or physical side effects of treatment, it's not necessary to unduly restrict all activity.

SEXUALITY

Although few people admit it, the fear that cancer is contagious still lurks. Nowhere does this fear have greater impact than in sexual relationships. All too often, the sex act is viewed as a possible vehicle for transmitting the disease. Women will ask if their husbands' prostate cancer could infect them through sexual intercourse. Husbands will worry that their wives' uterine cancer could infect them in the same way. If you have had these fears, you are by no means alone. However, there is no evidence to date that cancer is in any way contagious. In other words, it can't be sexually transmitted.

As with exercise and diet, patients are the best judges of how much sexual activity they feel like engaging in. Some cancer patients will be bedridden and nearly disabled, and therefore sexual activity will not be appealing or even possible. On the other hand, some people will feel relatively well, at least some of the time. They may desire this kind of intimacy and consider it part of living as fully as they can. Remember, however, that sexual intimacy need not involve intercourse. Touching, hugging, and so forth, are also part of intimacy.

We know that self-image has an enormous impact on sexuality. The cancer patient is no different, and self-image can be quite fragile. Those around him or her must be sensitive to this. Loss of a breast, loss of hair, and other visible damage to the body can cause anxiety, not to mention the fear that these changes will mar sexual attractiveness. These fears are understandable, but they are often blown out of proportion. In many cases, support groups or individual counseling can help.

Anna Gomez, a 45-year-old woman, underwent partial mastectomy for cancer and was seeing me for postoperative radiation therapy. She was concerned about the cosmetic appearance of her breast, since a considerable amount of tissue had been removed. She was quite concerned that her husband would no longer find her sexually attractive. She told me her husband tried to reassure her, but that she thought he was just placating her. After finding a local breast-cancer support group through the American Cancer Society, she was able to regain her own self-esteem and resolve the sexual issue in her marriage. By the end of treatment, her body image was remarkably improved.

SEEKING HELP FOR APPEARANCE ISSUES

Even with improved surgical techniques and radiation technology, many patients must cope with changes in their bodies. Nowadays, there are many resources available to help cancer patients adjust to these physical changes. Support groups and the American Cancer Society can help you. For example, breast-cancer support groups offer advice about the emotional adjustment to losing a breast, the pros and cons of reconstructive surgery, specially designed clothing, and so on.

Both men and women have to make practical adjustments to such treatment side effects as hair loss, and your local chapter of the American Cancer Society can help you locate centers that specialize in advising cancer patients about appearance and cosmetic issues. While these are never easy issues, seeking help can make them easier to cope with.

MAKING ADJUSTMENTS

It is difficult to do more than generalize about lifestyle during radiation treatment and recovery from cancer. There is simply too much individual variation among patients. And how a person feels has much to do with age, other medical conditions, and the severity of the disease.

When you have questions or concerns about your diet and other activities, ask your team of physicians and their staff to help you find the advice you need. Remember that you are in charge, and when you approach these issues with as positive an attitude as possible, you will feel better physically and emotionally.

Emotional Concerns

FOR MOST patients, having cancer also means experiencing an intense sense of isolation and a feeling of loneliness. Add the sense of dread that is invariably present, and an emotional situation is created that must be attended to. While all treatments for cancer have emotional ramifications, radiation treatment has an added component. The fear of the radiation itself, along with the attending side effects, even if mild, often exacerbates this most critical situation.

OVERCOMING FEAR OF TREATMENT

A recent patient of mine, Barbara Anderson, illustrates the kind of fear that can interfere with a person's quality of life during radiation treatment. Within a week of beginning her course of treatment, following the removal of an intestinal tumor, she began complaining of pain in both wrists. No amount of reassurance convinced her that the cancer had not spread to the bones in her wrists. (In fact, this would have been an extraordinarily rare occurrence.)

The only way I could alleviate Mrs. Anderson's fear was to x-ray her wrists and even perform a nuclear bone scan, both of which are diagnostic tests. When the results indicated that her bones were perfectly fine, her pain quickly subsided. Later she realized she had actually strained her wrists when she had enthusiastically tackled some household chores she had not felt up to doing before. Although diagnostic tests may have been unnecessary for *medical* reasons, they were crucial to her emotional well-being.

Pete Cowan, another patient, became depressed because he had misconceptions about radiation. One Monday morning he appeared quite despondent when he came in for his treatment for lung cancer. When I asked him how he felt, he told me it hurt him terribly to spend a weekend with his grandchildren but not be able to hug them or touch them in any way.

Mr. Cowan had assumed that he would contaminate others with his radioactivity because he believed that his body tissues were being transformed into dangerous radioactive material. Fortunately, I was able to reassure him that radiation delivered to the body is instantaneously changed to a biochemical state. Therefore, he posed no danger to anyone around him—and never would. The next day he was jubilant. Following our talk, he went to his daughter's house to spend some time with his grandchildren, this time without fear.

I have found that providing patients with the facts is the best way to help them overcome their fear of radiation treatment. This book may put many of your fears to rest. However, if you, like Mrs. Anderson, believe that other problems might arise from treatment, make sure that your physician is aware of your concerns and adequately addresses them. The fears that people express range from concern that the treatment is painless and silent and therefore "not working" to a worry that radiation will harm those around them.

KEEPING UP YOUR EMOTIONAL STRENGTH

Nearly all patients undergoing treatment for cancer experience some depression. It can be difficult to get the attention you need when you report depression to physicians and even to mental-health-care professionals. You might be told that it's normal to feel depressed when you are fighting cancer. This is true, but that doesn't make your depression any less valid.

Continue to talk with those involved in your care about your state of mind. While it is possible that the depression you are experiencing can be alleviated with medication, you may want to talk with a psychotherapist to help you through this difficult period when you may also be trying to accept the reality of your disease. Anger, denial, and sometimes the sense that the cancer is a punishment in some way are also emotional components of cancer. Therefore, it can be extremely helpful to seek information and emotional support from professionals, cancer self-help and support groups, and family members.

How a patient feels physically during the course of treatment is greatly affected by his or her emotional state. This can't be emphasized enough. Therefore, I recommend that cancer patients and their families ask their physicians about psychological support, generally available through the hospital, community centers, or other service agencies.

The American Cancer Society, for example, sponsors numerous programs and services for cancer patients, family members, and others. This well-known organization has extensive referral services linking those in need of help with the appropriate agencies. Some of the programs are based on the assumption that others who have had cancer can offer the best kind of support and understanding. I strongly recommend searching for programs that meet your individual needs and desires.

There are patients who, for a variety of reasons, don't feel comfortable participating in support groups, yet do want some emotional help. For these people I recommend regular counseling sessions with a therapist or, if that's not possible or appealing, with a spiritual counselor with whom they feel comfortable. Working with a counselor should be considered part of a total treatment plan. The goal is for you and those close to you to be able to cope with the facts of your illness in the most positive way possible.

Family members and friends may need their own support systems. Cancer can put great stress on families, and while some seem to pull closer together, other families are torn apart. If you are able to discuss this additional stress with your physicians, they may be able to guide you to appropriate help. Obviously, they can't interfere in your personal interactions, but providing support for the patient is an essential part of the physician's role. You should feel free to ask for advice and referrals.

MAINTAINING A POSITIVE ATTITUDE

Almost all patients and family members ask, "How important is a positive attitude?" I always respond, "Extremely important," but I know that this is sometimes easier said than done. Obviously, attitudes toward having cancer and being treated with radiation will vary greatly from person to person. Some people are more naturally optimistic than others. However, every cancer patient will need extra attention and support no matter how cheerful and positive he or she might seem.

Patients who understand their illness and their treatments become more active participants. The sense of helplessness and panic that accompanies a diagnosis of cancer may be reduced. Not only will these patients tend to have more rapid recovery from the side effects of treatment, but they may also better comply with treatment and have an improved health outcome.

Sometimes a patient will confuse the idea of being optimistic and gaining a sense of control over the illness with a denial of reality. This book certainly doesn't mean to encourage false cheerfulness or a pretense that the disease doesn't exist. In fact, a crucial step in reaching an optimistic attitude is dealing with the anger and the depression that invariably accompanies cancer. This usually requires the help and support of family, friends, support groups, or professional counseling. The people who experience the fewest debilitating side effects are often those who have confronted their fear and the reality of the disease. Furthermore, no cancer patient can be expected to be cheerful all the time. Those close to the patient will experience their own shifts in attitude too.

Having cancer can sometimes be a catalyst for much-needed change in a person's life. Tony Parker, a man whose lung cancer was discovered in its early stage, was such a person. After his first radiation treatment, he seemed to need enormous amounts of sleep. In fact, he slept most of the day and then stayed up during

the night watching television and dozing. He literally did nothing else, even refusing visits from family and friends.

Mr. Parker's wife and daughter were understandably upset
by this isolation and his withdrawn behavior. After a few office
visits he even walked with a stoop and shuffled along like a man
30 years older. In addition, he appeared somewhat disoriented. I
knew because of extensive prior testing that there was no physical reason for this behavior.

It was clear to me that Mr. Parker was suffering severe
emotional problems. His wife and daughter confirmed my suspi-
cions that he had been a relatively passive and dependent person
all his life. Having cancer simply allowed him to deepen his
dependence and let go of all responsibility. In turn, his wife and
daughter felt as if they were taking care of a baby. I referred him
to a psychiatrist who was able to help him change his attitude
and regain some sense of control over his life.

Francine Jones, a woman in her 40s with advanced lymphoma of the brain, spinal cord, and underarm area, received
radiation therapy to all these areas. She then reacted to her cancer by gathering all her strength and courage and remaining optimistic. Some people are remarkable in their ability to seemingly
beat the odds. In Ms. Jones's case, the outlook for even short-
term survival was guarded. In addition, she received chemotherapy concurrently with and following radiation treatment.

This woman's optimistic can-do personality served her well
during the course of her treatments. She read all the available
information about her illness, asked specific questions, listened
to relaxation tapes, and practiced self-help healing techniques. It
seemed like a miracle, but Ms. Jones was back to work within
two months. She coped with her side effects beautifully, and
when I talked with her two years later, she was doing quite well.

THE TRUTH IS ESSENTIAL

Most physicians and psychologists agree that a cancer patient
who is cheerful and optimistic does better than one who is negative and pessimistic. Since ancient times, health-care

professionals have talked about the will to live and its importance in recovery. However, in recent years research offers scientific evidence that a positive outlook may have measurable effect
on the course of cancer.

I believe it's virtually impossible for a patient to develop a
healthy optimism without knowing the facts. Therefore, I thoroughly describe the cancer to the patient—its origin, location,
and stage of aggressiveness. I also explain the chemical tests and
show the patient the x-ray and other imaging tests. This goes a
long way toward alleviating the fear of the unknown.
Furthermore, patients can then begin to have a sense of control
over their own condition. If cancer patients don't have a sense of
participation, the only alternative is feeling like helpless
observers or even victims.

The discussion about the cancer can be frank, but it need
not be brutal. Beating the "odds," no matter how grim, is always
a possibility. Some patients considered incurable not only have
outlived their prognosis, but have gone on to be cured.

Several things can contribute to a patient's positive attitude. Years ago, some physicians and lay people believed that
hiding or withholding information from a patient was beneficial,
but today we know better. What patients *don't* know may most
certainly hurt them. We also know that in the past, many cancer
patients did, in fact, realize how serious their conditions were.
But because others weren't talking openly, they, too, kept this
code of silence.

The code of silence might have been well intentioned, but
it led to a harmful emotional dishonesty between doctor and
patient. It was impossible to have an open relationship with a
cancer patient if information was withheld. Over the long run, I
believe that this resulted in anger, distrust, and probably
increased anxiety, because some patients became increasingly
isolated and had no one to talk with openly. Today's philosophy
of openness is sometimes difficult for patients to accept at first,
when they are just beginning to absorb the reality of their disease. However, it is clear that when honesty prevails, a trustful
relationship can develop, and patients can participate and maintain control over their treatment.

Occasionally I will violate my own rule about being completely open and honest with a patient. I was once concerned
that an 80-year-old man with cancer in multiple sites was too
frail to deal with the brutal facts of his illness. Therefore, I
became evasive and overemphasized the individual variation in
survival rates, painting too rosy a picture. He, however, was not
very tolerant of being protected. He became angry, rose out of
his chair, and yelled, "Stop treating me like a simpleton. Tell me
the truth!"

After I told this patient the *realistic* prognosis of his case, he
visibly relaxed and thanked me for being honest with him. He
also told me that he had demanded straight answers all his life,
and my evasiveness betrayed a trust he and I had developed.
Once I realized how strongly he felt, I was glad he had confronted
me with my mistake.

IMAGING: A SELF-HELP TECHNIQUE

One reason that cancer patients should know the facts about the
disease is that this information gives them an ability to actually
form an image of their fight against the cancer. These visualization techniques can have an effect on the eventual outcome of
cancer, and most certainly they have an impact on the way a person copes throughout the course of the illness.

The most important contribution to this body of work has
been made by Carl O. Simonton, M.D., a radiation oncologist
and a teacher. Written with his former wife, psychologist
Stephanie Simonton, *Getting Well Again* is one of my favorite
books about the interrelationship between mind and body.
There is no doubt that the Simontons' work has brought to the
public eye the importance of positive mental attitude in cancer
treatment.

Getting Well Again explains how cancer patients have tradi-
tionally assumed the role of passive bystander when confronted
with their disease. However, the Simontons found through their
work at the Cancer Counseling Center in Texas that conventional treatments are more effective when the patient takes an

active role and becomes a *partner* with physicians and their treatment team. Furthermore, the techniques the Simontons present may also alleviate physical pain and suffering and prolong life, even when a cure is not effected.

Dr. Simonton teaches a particular technique that uses visualization as a way of marshaling the body's immune system to fight the invading cancer cells. These imaging techniques, often referred to as guided imagery, include relaxation exercises which can be very beneficial in and of themselves. Some patients join self-help groups that practice the imaging and relaxation techniques, thereby offering additional support and understanding from others in similar circumstances.

Much of the Simontons' clinical success has been supported by recent research on the chemistry of the brain. We can now demonstrate that the mind is a major participant in the immune system, the body's system for protecting itself and fighting off invading disease. The imaging techniques appear to boost the immune system and enable the body to attack cancer. We now know that the body's natural defense system has a subtle and delicate relationship with brain chemistry. This knowledge is important in treating many diseases, cancer being one.

ANOTHER MEANINGFUL TOOL

Another book I recommend reading is *Love, Medicine and Miracles* by Bernie Siegal, M.D., a cancer surgeon. Dr. Siegal became fascinated by patients who seemingly cured themselves, and he wanted to discover how and why this happens. What he found, and reports in his book, is that patients who are able to deal with their anger and frustration quickly and move on to a more positive attitude increase their chances of beating the illness. His book is filled with numerous examples of people who took control of their lives and were even able to find humor and joy in themselves and their life situations.

The one component that appears to be crucial in facilitating not only a good outcome of the disease, but peace of mind, is love. It can't be emphasized enough that the loving relationships people have with those around them are of utmost importance when facing cancer. Siegal believes that if a patient is having conflicts with loved ones, or is still carrying around anger and resentment from the past, then healing those wounds should be a priority. Siegal also believes that a loving and trusting relationship between patients and their physicians is of vital importance. My own experience certainly bears this out.

One of my medical colleagues and friends developed lung cancer 10 years ago. His situation was very serious, and after surgery he underwent radiation therapy in my office. Ten years later he is in excellent condition. Recently I asked him to what he attributed his full recovery. He frankly admitted to me that he had absolutely no idea, but surmised it was probably due to his strong immune system. As my friend was talking, I watched his face and eyes, and I realized that for as long as I'd known him, he'd *always* seemed to have a smile on his face and a twinkle in his eye. His perpetual cheerfulness and positive outlook were characteristic of his personality. It was well known that this doctor was good for a new joke each week and had his listeners in uproarious laughter. In fact, there was no need to pursue the matter further—my colleague's face told the whole story.

Bernie Siegal affirms the power of love, not just for people who are ill, but for all of us who are trying to stay healthy. We can use this power if we are able to express our own emotional needs and behave in a loving manner with others. While this sounds simple, we know that it isn't necessarily easy to live this way. Sometimes an illness can show us how important it is to examine our lives and learn to give and receive love.

WHEN TREATMENT ENDS

Some patients see the end of a course of radiation therapy as a kind of "graduation day." They are glad to be finished with the daily obligation of treatment. However, a few patients become anxious as they near the end of therapy. They had a sense that as long as treatment continued, *something* was being done to combat the cancer. When treatment is over, they may feel a letdown.

If this happens to you, don't think you are abnormal; your feelings are understandable. Talk about them with your physicians, family members, friends, or others who are part of your support network.

The goal of emotional support is to bring a person to an acceptance of the reality of the disease without being thoroughly defeated by it. The two books mentioned above are certainly recommended to help you and your family members openly talk about how you are feeling and help you come to terms with the illness. Other books that may help you deal with emotional concerns are listed in the back of this book.

Cancer Treatment and Radiation Therapy

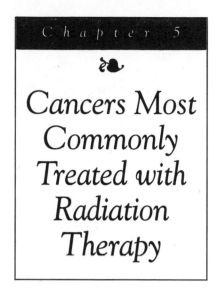

Cancers Most Commonly Treated with Radiation Therapy

PART 2 of this book is designed to give you information about specific cancer sites. However, it is wise to read part 1 first in order to have a general understanding of the purpose and process of radiation therapy. This chapter explains radiation treatment for the most commonly occurring cancers and the control of side effects for the specific area being treated. Subsequent chapters discuss treatment for sites where cancer has spread and ways in which pain can be managed or alleviated. I have also included a general discussion of chemotherapy. Many cancer patients are given chemotherapy before or after radiation treatments—some patients have chemotherapy and radiation treatments concurrently.

The cancers discussed below are those in which radiation therapy is likely to be recommended. Certain cancers—ovarian, liver, kidney, stomach, and the leukemias—are not usually treated with radiation therapy, but exceptions do occur. Childhood cancers are not discussed because the types of cancers that affect children are not often found in adults. Furthermore, most children are treated in special centers that are equipped to handle the unique medical and emotional concerns associated with childhood cancers.

The following sections are listed according to cancer site. *They are designed to provide a foundation of knowledge that you can use when discussing your specific case with your team of physicians. Dosages and times will vary among treatment centers and according to the patient's clinical picture. Your radiation therapist may recommend a different dosage of radiation, delivered over a different period of time. He or she may prescribe medications other than those I have cited and may suggest different alterations in lifestyle as well. Your own team of physicians will have very good reasons for the advice they offer. The information I'm providing is intended to serve as a guideline to radiation therapy, but is not a substitute for the individualized care you will receive.*

CANCER SITES (LISTED ALPHABETICALLY)

Bladder

In the early stages, bladder cancer is confined to the lining of that organ. The cancer is considered moderately advanced when it has spread from the lining to the underlying muscle of the bladder and the adjacent lymph nodes. (Human beings have thousands of lymph nodes, which act as biological filters that trap elements that are foreign to the body—infections or cancer, for example. Because lymph nodes are so widely distributed throughout the body, they are often affected when cancer spreads from its original site to adjacent tissues.) Cancer of the bladder is most advanced when it has invaded neighboring organs or has spread to distant organs such as the liver or the lungs.

TREATMENT. Early-stage bladder cancer is treated by surgically removing the tumor. Sometimes more than one area of the bladder is affected and multiple tumors are removed. Moderately advanced cancers are usually treated by surgery alone, radiation alone, or a combination of the two. Recently, chemotherapy has been used with radiation, a combination that has shown some promise for controlling this cancer in the future.

Complete removal of the bladder (cystectomy) or complete removal of the bladder with adjacent tissue and lymph nodes (radical cystectomy) are both commonly performed in the United States for moderately advanced bladder cancers. However, extensive studies in Europe have shown that these cancers respond as well with radiation alone or in combination with less radical surgery.

Significant long-term side effects and significantly high death rates are associated with treating bladder cancer with surgery alone. Both men and women who have had their bladder removed must have the ureters, the tubes leading from the kidneys to the bladder, implanted into the skin of the abdominal wall with an ostomy bag. Furthermore, men will become impotent as a result of the surgery. There are honest differences of opinion about the best way to treat bladder cancers, but after reviewing evidence for many years, I agree with the group that favors a combination of treatments.

Many radiation therapists prefer to preserve the bladder by performing high-dose radiation therapy. A total of 6,000 to 7,000 units of radiation may be delivered to the bladder and surrounding lymph nodes on a daily basis over a seven-week period. Treatment is directed through the front, back, and sides of the patient, or a rotational technique may be used, in which the machine rotates around the patient. Either technique is satisfactory.

I strongly believe in making every possible attempt to maintain the functional integrity of the bladder and, in men, the prostate as well. As long as the decision to keep the bladder intact does not influence the outcome for cure or control of the cancer, I believe that it is worthwhile to avoid radical surgery. Should radiation fail, the surgery can then be performed.

It appears that some patients have bladder cancers that are sensitive to radiation, while the disease of others is resistant. Those patients with radiation-sensitive tumors do not need surgery following radiation; those who show recurrence of the cancer within six months are considered radiation resistant, and may then undergo removal of the bladder.

Thus there is controversy about the best treatment of moderately advanced bladder cancer. Some patients are referred for preoperative radiation therapy to reduce the size of the tumor. Shrinking the size and the extent of the tumor often results in less radical surgery and also reduces operating time. Other patients receive radiation following surgery if the surgeon discovers that the tumor is more extensive than anticipated.

Patients whose cancers have advanced and invaded neighboring organs and those whose disease has spread to the lungs and liver receive palliative radiation. That is, the treatment is done to arrest the growth of the cancer and relieve symptoms. Radiation is given in moderate doses to control infection, obstruction, and bleeding caused by the tumor. Chemotherapy may also be used to control the cancer in distant sites, although this too has limited success.

SIDE EFFECTS. Radiation side effects can be minimized by allowing a month to pass between the bladder biopsy and the first treatment. Obstruction of the ureters caused by the cancer is treated by inserting tubes (Stents) to bypass the obstruction, and antibiotics are given to patients with bladder infections, which, while not common, can occur when the cancer is advanced.

In general, side effects during the six or seven weeks of radiation therapy are moderate. It is common for the bladder to become irritated and the patient to experience some urinary frequency, some burning, and urinary urgency, the latter being the urge to urinate even though the bladder is empty. These symptoms are well controlled with appropriate medications. (I prefer Pyridium or Ditropan.) Warm baths, especially prior to going to bed at night, are also helpful in reducing urinary urgency. The side effects must be distinguished from symptoms of urinary-tract infection (UTI), because bladder irritation caused by the radiation and an infection can mimic each other or coexist. Therefore, a urinalysis is done frequently so that an infection can be treated with antibiotics if it occurs. In such cases, the antibiotics are used with medications given to relieve bladder irritation.

Bowel symptoms may also be present, because radiation affects the rectum and the lower intestine. Patients will experience diarrhea, cramping, and an urge to evacuate even when no fecal material is present. (The latter is called tenesmus.) I recommend the medications Lomotil or Imodium A-D to relieve diarrhea and cramping.

Irritation in the rectal area may require a medication such as Anusol-HC suppositories or cream. Moderate reddening of the skin over the area receiving radiation, particularly between the folds of the buttocks, can be treated with skin creams such as Nivea or cortisone ointments. These and other symptoms can be controlled, and most patients are able to continue radiation treatments without major difficulty.

A minority of patients may have long-term side effects following radiation treatment. These include occasional bleeding from the bladder, known as hemorrhagic cystitis, and bladder contraction with decreased ability to retain urine. A few patients may develop an obstruction or bleeding from the small intestine.

FOLLOW-UP AND OUTLOOK. It is essential that following treatment, patients undergo periodic urologic examinations. Patients who have not had a cystectomy and have received only radiation therapy will receive follow-up cystoscopies and x-rays of the chest, IVPs, and CT scans of the pelvis (see chapter 9). A cystoscopy is a procedure in which the bladder is viewed through a special instrument in order to confirm that no new growths have appeared. Those patients who have had cystectomies will undergo CT scans for follow-up evaluation.

Clinical trials are currently being done to evaluate the results of surgery, radiation therapy, and combination treatment plans. Chemotherapeutic agents, particularly 5FU and cysplatin, are being tried in conjunction with radiation. Chemotherapy has been shown to enhance the effects of radiation therapy. More trials are needed to better determine the role of chemotherapy in future treatment of this type of cancer.

Brain

Radiation therapy is delivered to the brain either to treat a cancer originating there (a primary cancer) or, more commonly, for cancer that has spread (metastasized) from a distant site. To avoid confusion, each situation will be discussed separately. Treatment for cancer *originating* in the brain is discussed in this section; treatment for metastatic cancer of the brain is discussed in chapter 6.

CT scans and MRI scans (see chapter 9) are generally used to detect brain tumors. These tests enable neurosurgeons and radiation therapists to precisely locate the tumor and its extensions. Although tests are very sensitive, they are not specific, meaning that they also image conditions that mimic cancer. Therefore, if a primary brain cancer is suspected, a biopsy is usually required before a definitive diagnosis is made.

Surgery is used to confirm the diagnosis of cancer, determine the cell type, and reduce the size of the tumor by removing as much of the diseased tissue as possible. This is a very delicate procedure in which care is taken not to damage the surrounding normal structures. Radiation therapy is administered if the tumor has not been completely removed.

TREATMENT. Once surgery is completed and it is determined that the cell type is sensitive to radiation, radiation therapy is begun. Both CT and MRI scans are used to design an appropriate treatment field. If the tumor is the type that is very invasive, larger areas of the brain are treated. However, in many patients, the treatment portal includes only the area of known disease and some of the surrounding tissue. (Treatment for metastatic disease generally involves the whole brain.)

Depending on the location of the disease and its particular characteristics, radiation treatment may involve multiple portals through the front, back, or the sides of the head. A multiple-portal treatment plan maximizes the dose of radiation to the tumor, while minimizing the radiation that reaches normal tissue. In other words, the dosage of radiation must be adequate to fight the cancer but, as much as possible, spare the vital brain tissues.

Approximately 6,000 to 6,500 units are typical doses that may be delivered in seven weeks. We treat the anticipated route of extension of the tumor as well as the tumor that is visible at the time of diagnosis.

Treatments are generally given daily over a five- to seven-week period. The dose and length of the treatment course depends on the individual's clinical situation as well as his or her general physical health, the particular cell type of the tumor, and its location.

Recently, lymphoma in the brain has been on the increase. This special type of brain cancer was once considered an oddity. However, the immunosuppression associated with AIDS has led to a dramatic rise in incidence of non-Hodgkin's lymphoma of the brain. At this time, whole-brain radiation and cortisone medication are the standard treatments, and they are effective in 50 percent of cases. Unfortunately, the period of remission (arrest of the disease process) in patients who respond to treatment is usually brief (three to six months at best), and patients with AIDS-associated lymphoma of the brain may have disease in other organs as well.

Infectious disease of the brain may mimic AIDS-associated lymphoma, and therefore a biopsy is necessary to confirm an initial diagnosis. A total dose of 3,000 to 4,000 units of radiation, administered over a four- to five-week period, is usually necessary to alleviate symptoms in those patients who will respond to radiation treatment.

SIDE EFFECTS. To combat the immediate side effects of radiation therapy, patients are usually given two types of medication during the period when they are receiving radiation treatments. The first, a cortisone medication (Decadron or prednisone), reduces swelling (edema) in the brain tissues. This swelling may be caused by the tumor itself, or it may occur as a side effect of treatment. The second type of medication (Dilantin) is given to prevent convulsions.

One of the most psychologically troubling side effects of radiation therapy to the brain is hair loss. Most people are very concerned about this, because aesthetic or body-image issues invariably become emotional issues as well. Some patients do not experience significant hair loss because they have very strong hair follicles, a characteristic that is genetic and can't be changed. Most people, however, do lose the hair over the treated area, beginning two to three weeks into the treatment period. Because we know that hair loss is likely, I strongly recommend that patients arrange for a hairpiece when treatment begins. By doing so, they avoid a distressing period of noticeable baldness. Hair loss will continue throughout treatment and for several weeks after the radiation therapy course is completed.

Occasionally, the hair grows back, but the texture is altered and the growth is sparse. (When hair loss is associated with chemotherapy, the hair loss is not restricted to the head but may also affect all body hair.)

One to two hours after receiving a radiation treatment to the brain, it is common for patients to become drowsy and possibly slightly disoriented. Because this side effect is likely to occur, I advise patients to rest or sleep following treatment. Patients sometimes become alarmed by these symptoms, but there is no cause for concern. Both the drowsiness and the disorientation disappear within a few hours. Fatigue may begin at some time during the course of treatment.

Nausea is an infrequent side effect, but if it occurs, it can be well controlled with medication. (I prefer Compazine.) Following treatment, some patients experience mild headaches that can be treated with over-the-counter medications. The skin over the area of treatment also reddens because of the radiation irritation, and a skin cream such as Nivea is effective in relieving this symptom. These side effects may be annoying, but they are not serious.

Severe headaches, projectile vomiting (forceful vomiting), and visual changes occur infrequently, but they must be reported immediately. These symptoms may signal an increase in pressure, caused by the swelling within the brain. In some cases, it is necessary to temporarily interrupt treatments and increase the dosage of cortisone medication to reduce swelling.

Patients are understandably concerned about receiving radiation treatment to the brain. Any disease process going on in the brain is especially worrisome. After all, the brain is the organ that directs all of human activity. Our thoughts and emotions originate in the brain, and it is considered the center of the self. Therefore, I urge patients to get emotional support from family, friends, and also from professionals if possible. It is essential to call on all available support systems during these stressful times.

Unfortunately, delayed side effects of radiation to the brain include long-term changes in intellectual functioning and memory. However, many adults with brain tumors do not survive long enough to experience these effects, because many primary brain cancers are very aggressive and long-term survival rates are low.

FOLLOW-UP AND OUTLOOK. Chemotherapy has been used to increase survival time by several months. Current research is attempting to determine which drugs may yield better results than are obtained with those chemical agents being administered at the present time. Occasionally, radioactive pellets are implanted into the tumor, but there is no evidence that this offers additional chances for a cure. To date, radiation therapy and chemotherapy following surgery are the best treatment methods available.

Because many brain cancers are aggressive and advanced when discovered, cure rates are low. However, radiation therapy can improve symptoms and temporarily arrest the tumor growth. CT and MRI scans are performed one to two months following treatment and then periodically as part of routine follow-up care. However, if symptoms return, they are treated with appropriate medications in order to preserve as good a quality of life as possible.

Breast

Breast cancer usually arises from the milk-forming glandular structures (mammary ducts). It first spreads locally into the surrounding tissues. Then, after a variable period of time—months or sometimes years—it invades the lymph vessels, depositing itself in nearby lymph nodes. It may invade blood vessels (arteries and veins) thereby traveling to distant sites in the body (metastases).

TREATMENT. At the present time, there is considerable controversy surrounding the most appropriate treatment of this cancer, and each patient's treatment is individualized to her particular clinical situation. The treatment approaches described here are those that I and many cancer specialists and radiation therapists currently favor. However, these treatments may change in the future as more clinical data is acquired. The discussions about the best treatments are legitimate and important, and patients today have options that were at one time not available. Therefore, patients are encouraged to seek additional opinions about any treatment presented here.

In the past decade, breast cancer treatment has undergone significant modification. At one time, radical breast surgery, known as radical mastectomy, was considered the ideal treatment. This surgery included removal of the breast, the underlying muscles, and a large number of underarm lymph nodes. (Human beings have thousands of lymph nodes, which act as filters for elements foreign to the body—infection and cancer, for example. Because lymph nodes are so widely distributed throughout the body, they often are affected when cancer begins to spread from its original site to adjacent tissues.) After many clinical studies here and abroad, it was discovered that less radical surgery combined with radiation therapy was just as effective. Thus, a modified radical mastectomy involving removal of the breast but sparing the major muscles and reducing surgery to underarm lymph nodes, often followed by radiation therapy, yielded similar survival results.

Depending on the stage of the cancer, women may undergo total (also called simple) mastectomy, which removes the breast and spares all the underlying muscles, with limited surgery to lymph nodes. Radiation may also be recommended.

Mammography (See Chapter 9) has led to more diagnoses of breast cancer in its earliest stages. As a result, the surgical procedure known as lumpectomy (more formally referred to as breast conservation surgery) is now performed with greater frequency. The procedure involves removing the small tumor plus a generous margin of surrounding breast tissue. However, the breast itself is not removed. Many surgeons perform additional surgery to the underarm axillary areas in order to check the status of the lymph nodes, because these structures are usually the next area affected by the spread of the disease. Following surgery, radiation treatments are given to the affected breast and may also be administered to the adjacent lymph nodes.

This therapy following a lumpectomy is necessary because any nests of tumor cells, which may be present in the breast but are not detected manually or with mammography, will be destroyed by the radiation. The combination treatment, lumpectomy and radiation therapy, has been found to be as effective as mastectomy in preventing recurrence of the tumor in the local chest wall. The eventual possibility of developing distant metastases have been shown to be the same for both groups of patients. Therefore, the long term survival rates are virtually the same.

Many large studies of patients both in Europe and the United States, involving a total of more than 4000 women, have demonstrated these results. In 1990. the National Cancer Institute Consensus Development Conference on the treatment of early stage breast cancer declared breast conservation surgery and "appropriate method of primary therapy for the majority of women" with early stage breast cancer.

Those patients who undergo modified radical mastectomy and whose removed lymph nodes are free of cancer *do not* require radiation treatment. However, if lymph nodes are discovered to be positive for cancer in those patients requiring a modified radical mastectomy, postoperative radiation is administered because it is known to reduce recurrence of cancer in the chest wall and other lymph nodes. Usually 5,000 units are delivered in five-and-a-half to six weeks.

Not everyone is a candidate for lumpectomy. Those who may be include women with tumors measuring less that 5cm (2 inches) in size. This group consists of more than 50 percent of breast cancer patients. Prior to radiation therapy, it is important to perform a mammogram on the affected breast to make sure that all malignant calcifications have been removed. In addition, most current breast cancer patients have received either hormone therapy or chemotherapy before radiation treatments begin. (The sequencing of combined treatments is currently being investigated and therefore, protocols are undergoing rapid change.)

Most patients with large tumors of those who have *multiple* tumors in the breast should choose mastectomy. On a mammogram, multiple tumors usually appear as areas of abnormal calcifications throughout the breast. Incidence of recurrence of the cancer is high on these patients and therefore, a mastectomy, which removes all breast tissue, is recommended.

Pregnant women, who should not be exposed to radiation treatments, are also generally restricted to the mastectomy option. Women who have already received radiation to the chest area (to treat Hodgkin's disease, for example). or who have a disease affecting connective tissue ("lupus" or scleroderma) are also not considered candidates for radiation therapy because the tissues will not tolerate radiation treatments.

If the cancer recurs in patients who have undergone lumpectomy and radiation, it is usually detected with mammography, physical examination, or both. Mastectomy can then be performed with (as yet) no demonstrable change in overall survival statistics.

Surgery or radiation do not prevent the cancer from spreading to distant sites (metastases). It is currently thought that many women who eventually develop cancer in distant sites may have already had nondetectable cancer in these sites at the time of their surgery and/or radiation. Therefore, modern chemical testing is attempting to increase the possibility of determining which patient groups might be at greatest risk for metastases. Many such tests are currently being used. Patients identified to be at high risk are given chemotherapy and hormonal therapy in an attempt to reduce the growth of the cancer in these distant metastases.

Radiation treatment plans include delivering radiation to all the local lymph-node groups. It is also delivered to the chest wall if, at the time of surgery, many nodes are found to harbor cancer. If the breast is still in place, then treatment is delivered to the breast itself, and sometimes to the lymph nodes, depending on the woman's clinical situation. This treatment requires a high degree of accuracy, and a physicist often works with the radiation therapist to achieve maximum precision. Treatments are given on a daily basis for five to seven weeks, for a total of 6,500 units. I prefer 5,000 units to the whole breast, followed by a "booster" dose to the lumpectomy site of 1,600 units.

Although all breast-cancer patients are at risk for having the cancer spread to distant sites, those women with known spread to the local lymph-node groups are particularly at risk. Thus, chemotherapeutic drugs may be given even when *no known* cancer is left following surgery and radiation. This is called *adjuvant* chemotherapy. Currently, a combination of cyclophosphamide, methotrexate, and fluorouracil (CMF) is commonly given to premenopausal women. An antihormonal agent, Nolvadex (a brand name of tamoxifen), may also be used, particularly for postmenopausal women. The drug blocks the stimulating effect on the tumor of the female hormone, estrogen. Tamoxifen and radiation do not interact with each other, and therefore, side effects of either treatment are not exacerbated by the other. In addition, chemotherapy and radiation treatments are generally not administered concurrently, and the side effects of each treatment can be managed separately. When it is given, chemotherapy usually precedes radiation therapy by several months.

The factors that currently determine the use of these drugs include the number of axillary lymph nodes that are positive for cancer, the size of the primary cancer, the woman's age (pre- or postmenopausal), and the sensitivity of the cancer cells to estrogen and progesterone. The latter is determined at the time the tumor is removed by means of a special laboratory test.

Clinical trials are currently being performed to see if patients with *no* evidence of cancer in the lymph nodes can benefit from drug therapy. In other words, these studies are attempting to determine if all breast cancer patients should be placed on some form of medication. Because a variety of chemotherapeutic agents are constantly being reevaluated, today's guidelines will change in the future as more information is gathered and analyzed.

SIDE EFFECTS. Side effects of radiation therapy to the breast include some moderate skin reddening over the breast. A mild rash, which sometimes blisters or cracks, may occasionally occur in the sensitive underarm area. The symptoms are relieved and the skin condition is reversed with skin creams (I prefer Nivea) and cortisone preparations.

Nowadays, because of modern super voltage machines, the side effects to the skin are generally not very troublesome and can be compared to a mild sunburnlike reddening. Fair-skinned women generally experience more skin reactions than those with darker skin. Like a sunburn, the darkened area will gradually peel and return to its normal shade in a few months. Talcum powder can relieve itching that may occur when the skin is peeling.

Occasionally, patients may complain of a slight difficulty in swallowing if the radiation needs to be directed to lymph nodes behind the breast bone. Avoiding hot or cold foods and taking liquid antacids generally alleviate these symptoms, which are caused by the radiation irritation of the esophagus.

Women who have had lumpectomies followed by radiation to the affected breast often complain of soreness, tenderness, or pain in the remaining breast tissue. These symptoms can be relieved by applying warm-water compresses during the course of treatment. This discomfort promptly disappears when the therapy is completed, and generally this soreness is more of an inconvenience than a problem. When fatigue is present, it is usually mild.

Many women do not experience any significant side effects while under treatment, and most symptoms are reported as annoying rather than serious. For the most part, these patients are able to carry on normal schedules and lead their usual lifestyles.

Some patients (about 10 percent) who have had surgery in the underarm area to evaluate lymph nodes will develop some swelling in the affected arm. This can be minimized with exercises, such as squeezing a ball or "walking" that arm up a wall.

In addition to the immediate side effects described above, there may be some *long term* changes. In some women, the skin of the treated breast may permanently thicken; in others, it may become thin. There may also be some depigmentation of the nipple and adjacent tissue. There will be some internal scarring of the breast, which may create firmness in the tissue and a slight reduction in breast size.

Many women do not experience any side effects *while under treatment* and most symptoms are reported as annoying rather than serious. For the most part, patients are able to maintain their usual schedules and lead their normal lifestyles.

The emotional component may be a troublesome aspect of breast-cancer treatment. Many women feel a great loss of sexual appeal, and their self-image may be damaged by either the partial or total loss of a breast. The lumpectomy has greatly alleviated this reaction, but it may still be present. In addition, women are anxious both during and following treatment because they are not considered free of the disease for approximately 10 years. Most of the *meaningful* statistics on breast-cancer survival and lack of recurrence are based on the 10-year experience rather than the conventional 5-year observation. As a result, there is a natural anxiety about the eventual outcome. Because she is always at risk, a woman always feels "special" in some way. It is an unfortunate situation that, at this point, can't be changed.

Nowadays, there are excellent support groups for women with breast cancer. The American Cancer Society sponsors a self-help group called Reach to Recovery. Volunteers who have had breast cancer help other women cope with the fear, anger, sadness, and other emotions that invariably accompany this illness. Husbands and partners should also become involved. I strongly recommend becoming involved with self-help groups. They have been of great value to many of my patients because these groups provide psychological support both during and after treatment.

FOLLOW-UP AND OUTLOOK. Because of the nature of breast cancer, it is absolutely essential that women have periodic follow-up examinations. These tests include mammography, nuclear bone scans and bone x-rays if bone pain develops, chest x-rays and CT scans (see chapter 9) according to symptoms, and appropriate blood tests. These tests are performed routinely over the decade following the initial treatment.

Currently, it is recommended that the breast treated with lumpectomy and radiation should be physically examined and mammogrammed every six months for a period of three years, a schedule that starts approximately eight months after completion of radiation therapy. These frequent mammograms are recommended so that any changes in the breast, which could indicate recurrence of the cancer, can be detected as early as possible. After three years, annual mammograms are recommended. The opposite breast should be examined with an annual mammogram because it is at a higher risk for developing cancer. This is also true for women who have undergone mastectomy.

With the increasing use of mammography for screening purposes, more and more cancers will be detected in the early stages. This has already been proven by the many screening studies performed. I have served as assistant director of a nationwide screening study at the New Jersey College of Medicine and

Dentistry in which we detected breast cancers the size of a pin-head with mammography, long before they could be felt through manual examination. Thus, there are increasing numbers of patients who are, or should be, undergoing minimal surgery followed by radiation therapy.

To date, treatment results still depend greatly on the stage at which breast cancer has been discovered. Cure rates are much better when a woman has a small tumor (usually diagnosed by mammography) and no tumor in the lymph nodes than when lymph nodes are found to contain cancer. (It has recently been reported in medical literature that the treatment protocol consisting of lumpectomy followed by radiation therapy is not being offered as an option as often as it should be. The modified radical mastectomy is still being favored, even though the lumpectomy-and-radiation combination treatment has been endorsed by the National Cancer Institute. Patients must demand that all options be presented and thoroughly discussed before they make treatment choices.) The long term effects of radiation therapy to the breast after lumpectomy have yet to be determined.

Cervix

The cervix is the lower portion of the uterus, and it connects that organ with the vagina. Cervical cancer is biologically different from that occurring in the rest of the uterus and is therefore discussed separately. Nowadays, cancer of the cervix can often be detected in its early stages because we have the Pap smear available as a diagnostic tool. This test allows cells that are shed by the cervix to be analyzed for the presence of cancer. There is a cause-and-effect relationship between cervical cancer and sexually transmitted diseases, which are now on the rise. Therefore, it is possible that we will see an increase in cervical cancer.

TREATMENT. Treatment for this condition is very individualized, because many treatment options are available depending on the total clinical situation. In its early stage, the treatment of cervical cancer is not complex. Localized surgery to remove the area affected by the cancer is usually all that is necessary. (Fertility is not affected.) When more of the cervix is involved, the uterus, the fallopian tubes, and sometimes the ovaries are removed.

When cancer spreads beyond the cervix, the lymph nodes in the pelvis and upper vagina are frequently affected and radiation therapy is the usual treatment. (The human body has thousands of lymph nodes whose function is to filter elements that are foreign to the body—infection and cancer, for example. Because they are so widely distributed throughout the body, lymph nodes are often affected when cancer spreads beyond its original site.)

Radiation treatments may be both external and internal. External radiation is delivered to the outside of the body in the conventional manner. Internal radiation (brachytherapy) consists of placing radioactive material, commonly referred to as *sources*, in the vagina. The decision to use one or the other method of radiation is based on each patient's clinical situation. Patients who are not considered candidates for surgery, or who have more advanced disease, are treated with a combination of external and internal radiation.

A total dose of 5,000 to 6,000 units of *external* radiation may be delivered in a five- to seven-week period. Treatment is delivered through portals to the front, the back, and the sides of the pelvis.

In the United States, the most often-used radioactive source for *internal* treatment of the cervix is cesium-137. The treatment is designed to deliver a very high dose of radiation to the local lymph nodes in the area of the cervix and the upper vagina. Internal radiation therapy is given in one or two applications, each lasting several days. The radioactive source is usually inserted in the cervix and the uterus while the woman is under anesthesia. Therefore, she is hospitalized and confined to total bed rest during the time that the radioactive source is in place.

The radioactive material is very powerful and lethal to the cancer cells. However, some of the radioactive energy escapes beyond the body and is considered a potential hazard to others if exposure is prolonged. Therefore, every hospital takes precautions to minimize this potential risk, thus insuring the safety of visitors and hospital staff. In essence, this results in isolation of the patient except for necessary visits by health-care providers.

Quite recently, an alternate method of administering internal radiation has been introduced in the United States, although it has already gained wide popularity in Europe and Asia. The method involves inserting the radioactive sources in rapid high doses. The treatment is delivered on an outpatient basis, thus avoiding the complications and cost associated with general anesthetic and a hospital stay. Satisfactory results have been achieved with five treatments, which are combined with external radiation therapy. It has been demonstrated that this rapid, high-dose method is as effective as the traditional low-dose treatment previously described. However, it involves extensive technical and nursing support staff.

SIDE EFFECTS. Diarrhea and urinary frequency usually occur two to three weeks into treatment. The diarrhea can be treated with medications such as Lomotil and Imodium A-D; urinary frequency is treated with medications such as Pyridium and Ditropan. Irritation of the skin over the area receiving radiation can be treated with skin creams (I generally prefer Nivea) and cortisone ointments.

When radiation is the only treatment, high doses are required, and long-term (chronic) side effects may result. Intestinal side effects include rectal irritation and ulcers, and sometimes a narrowing of the bowel with some accompanying obstruction. Chronic bladder inflammation and narrowing of the outlet to the bladder are also possible, and there will be a narrowing of the vagina because of scarring of the tissues. When radiation and surgery are used in combination, the severity of side effects is decreased.

The highest incidence of cervical cancer occurs among women 45 to 55 years old. There is often a considerable emotional component in treatment decisions because it is possible that radiation treatment will affect sexual functioning. If cervical cancer has spread to the uterus, necessitating its removal, the loss of the uterus may be perceived as a loss of sexuality. This is more pronounced in women of childbearing age if pregnancy was desired in the future. In addition, some of the delayed side effects of radiation may include vaginal scarring with accompanying sexual dysfunction because the vaginal tissues may lose elasticity—the ability to stretch. Most women seek psychological counseling to cope with this problem, and some women may need surgical procedures to counteract the effects of the scarring. In order to minimize the effects of lost elasticity, the vaginal tissues may need periodic stretching.

FOLLOW-UP AND OUTLOOK. Regular follow-up with a gynecologist is essential. Currently, researchers are investigating the role of adjuvant chemotherapy (chemical treatment when no known disease is left) to determine if it can prevent recurrence. However, to date, the best hope for curing cervical cancer lies in its early detection through routine gynecological exams, including Pap smears.

Colon (Lower Intestine)

Cancer of the colon usually develops in the tissues that line the inner surfaces of the intestines. Undetected, it extends outward into the local intestinal muscle walls and then to surrounding tissues, lymph nodes, lymph vessels, and blood vessels.

TREATMENT. Surgery is the usual treatment for colon cancer. If the most distal part of the colon, the rectum, is involved, then a colostomy will be performed. This means that after the cancerous area has been removed, the remaining end of the colon is attached to the skin of the abdominal wall. There, the opening (stoma) is covered by a removable bag to catch fecal material. In all other locations of the colon, the cut ends are brought together without need for a colostomy, following removal of cancerous areas. For example, the sigmoid colon, a portion of the colon adjacent to the rectum, frequently affected by cancer, may not require a colostomy as part of the treatment plan.

Before surgery, various diagnostic tests are performed to evaluate the extent of the disease. These consist primarily of a chest x-ray, abdominal and pelvic CT scans, and ultrasound examinations. These are done to see if the cancer has spread to other organs. The liver, the lung, and abdominal lymph nodes are the most common sites of spread.

Radiation therapy may be used following surgery for rectal and sigmoid cancers when these cancers have invaded the neighboring tissues. The purpose of radiation therapy is to treat lymph nodes and tissues surrounding the colon which are known to contain cancer cells or are suspected of harboring remaining cancer cells. (Lymph nodes act as filters for elements foreign to the body—infection and cancer, for example. We have thousands of lymph nodes located throughout the body, and therefore, they are often affected when cancer begins to spread from its original site to adjacent tissues.) Radiation therapy is thought to be effective in destroying cells in the neighboring nodes and tissues, thus reducing the chances of the cancer's recurring in the pelvic area.

Part of the radiation therapy may be delivered *before* surgery if the cancer originates in the rectum or sigmoid colon. This sequence has often improved chances for survival because it frequently shrinks the cancer, thereby making it more operable. (When the cancer occurs in parts of the colon other than the rectum or the sigmoid colon, preoperative radiation therapy has not been shown to be effective.) Following surgery, radiation therapy is then continued to higher dose levels to treat lymph nodes that may contain cancer. Some surgeons, however, prefer that their patients receive radiation therapy only *following* surgery if a tumor is discovered in the local tissues, because preoperative radiation therapy necessarily delays surgery. Some physicians consider this delay to be detrimental to the patient.

The radiation therapy plan, both pre- and postoperative, for colon cancer usually involves four portals (areas under treatment) aimed at the pelvic soft tissues and the lymph nodes. Usually, 4,000 to 5,000 units are given over four to six weeks *post*operatively; the average length of treatment is about five weeks. *Pre*operative radiation treatment schedules vary widely. Some cancer specialists favor a short course of high-dose treatments; others prefer 4,500 units in five weeks. Patients may be given chemotherapy at the same time that radiation therapy is administered. Sometimes chemotherapy follows a course of radiation treatment. We do know that chemotherapy (5FU) may actually enhance the effectiveness of radiation therapy by sensitizing the cancerous tissue to radiation. However, chemotherapy will also aggravate the side effects of radiation. Often, drugs to stimulate the immune system are also given with chemotherapy.

SIDE EFFECTS. The most common side effects of radiation to the colon are cramping and diarrhea, usually appearing toward the end of the second week and early in the third week of treat-ment. As with other side effects, there is great variation in severity among individual patients. Fortunately, these symptoms are easily controlled with medications such as Lomotil, Pepto-Bismol, or Imodium A-D. Patients who experience rectal irrita-tion are usually able to obtain relief with suppositories. (I prefer Anusol-HC.)

Although dosages of medications are gradually reduced dur-ing treatment as symptoms subside, I find that it is best for patients to stay on some medication throughout the entire course of radiation treatment once the diarrhea and cramping begin. If symptoms are present when the treatment is complete, I advise patients to continue the medication for another week or two. Persistent symptoms warrant barium tests (see chapter 9) or colonoscopy, because the symptoms may be caused by underlying medical conditions such as colitis or diverticulosis.

The medications that relieve the gastrointestinal side effects work best when combined with dietary modifications. In addition, I am convinced that the changes in diet may allow the dosages of medications to be reduced. Generally, patients feel best on a low-fat diet that also excludes raw fruits and vegetables. All foods and beverages must be decaffeinated (see chapter 3).

At about the same time, or shortly after the gastrointestinal symptoms begin, most patients experience urinary frequency and urgency. They may feel the need to urinate but pass only small amounts of water. Again, good results are usually achieved with available medications. (I prefer Pyridium or Ditropan.) Before the medication is given, however, a urinary-tract infection (UTI) must be ruled out, because the symptoms are the same. If an infection is present, antibiotics are administered. (People with a prior history of urinary-tract infections have an increased chance of developing a UTI during treatment.) Immersing in a warm bath once or twice a day, particularly before going to bed, also helps alleviate urinary urgency and frequency.

Toward the end of treatment (four to five weeks) patients may complain of irritation between the folds of the buttocks and in the rectal area. Cortisone creams are effective in eliminating discomfort, usually within a few days.

Many patients experience considerable fatigue toward the end of treatment when radiation therapy is administered to the pelvic region. Because this is a common symptom in many radiation treatment programs, I always tell my patients about this side effect before they begin their treatment.

The fatigue that people feel may have nothing to do with the disease process but is caused by what used to be called *radiation sickness*. The fatigue appears to be caused by the chemicals released as the cancer cells are destroyed, although this is not fully documented. These products circulate in the bloodstream and are perceived by the body as toxins. This run-down feeling is similar to that experienced by people with chronic infections, and the mechanisms that produce the fatigue are probably the same. It should be emphasized that the severity of the fatigue varies greatly among individuals. Although this variation may, in part, be caused by a person's natural resistance, it is also very much due to the size of the tumor and the consequent volume of "breakdown products" as radiation therapy destroys cancer cells. The majority of patients have recovered from the fatigue when they return for follow-up visits two to three weeks after radiation therapy is completed.

Unfortunately, not much can be done to counter the fatigue syndrome except to offer the realistic reassurance that, in most cases, this goes away fairly rapidly. Those patients who are receiving chemotherapy during the radiation therapy, or have received it prior to radiation, may find their fatigue to be even more pronounced. However, it is important to understand that most fatigue experienced while receiving radiation therapy is not caused by cancer activity. As previously noted, this side effect may be aggravated by chemotherapy.

By and large, most patients are able to continue their usual lifestyles. Employed people often manage to continue working right through the entire course of treatment. It is safe to say that younger people, with no underlying medical conditions in addition to the cancer, generally tolerate the fatigue associated with radiation therapy more easily than do older individuals. In addition, emotional factors profoundly influence the person's perception of fatigue. For example, excessive anxiety significantly contributes to the feeling of fatigue.

FOLLOW-UP AND OUTLOOK. Following completion of the treatment course, patients are evaluated periodically to make sure that the cancer has not reactivated locally or spread to distant sites. Local spread of rectal or sigmoid cancer usually affects the lower area of the spine (the sacrum), and pain is often a symptom when this occurs. Spread to more distant sites, if it occurs, appears first in the liver and lymph nodes located near the liver. Occasionally, the lungs and brain are affected.

Because of the known routes of cancer spread, appropriate x-ray tests are obtained periodically. These include CT scans of the pelvis and abdomen to specifically evaluate the lymph nodes of the pelvis and abdomen as well as the liver. If a patient complains of pain or other problems in some specific place, then other diagnostic tests may be performed, such as an MRI scan of the brain, ultrasound examinations of the liver, bone x-rays, and nuclear bone scans (see chapter 9). Blood tests to evaluate liver function are also routinely done, since they may detect early metastatic disease before it is seen on CT scans. A specialized blood test, which measures a chemical known as CEA, also evaluates colon cancer activity. A rising level of CEA generally indicates colon cancer activity somewhere in the body, and can signal recurrence of the disease in its early stages. We then investigate further to locate the site of recurrence.

Colon cancer is one of the most common cancers in the United States, and it is reassuring to know that early detection significantly increases the chances for survival. Early detection tests include a rectal examination performed by a physician and the testing of stool for blood. (Commercial kits are available for self-testing). The best tests for colorectal cancers are barium enemas (see chapter 9) and colonoscopy. The latter involves the use of a flexible tube with a light so that the physician can directly view the lining of the lower intestine.

Esophagus

The esophagus is the narrow tube that allows food to pass from the throat down to the stomach. It begins in the neck, extends down into the chest, and ends in the upper abdomen at the level of the stomach. Cancer of the esophagus usually develops in the cells that line the organ's inner wall. Because the esophagus is narrow and has very thin walls, small cancers may quickly cause symptoms. A person notices that the passage of food and liquids is obstructed and generally seeks medical advice because of this change.

Unfortunately, cancer in the esophagus generally spreads rapidly and usually affects lymph nodes by the time it is detected. (The human body has thousands of lymph nodes, whose function is to filter elements that are foreign to the body—infections and cancer, for example. Because lymph nodes are so widely distributed throughout the body, they are often affected when cancer begins to spread from its original site to adjacent tissues.) The majority of patients who are diagnosed with cancer of the esophagus have extensive local disease or metastases to distant sites. Cure is generally not possible in these cases.

TREATMENT. Cancers in the upper and mid third of the esophagus generally respond better to radiation therapy; surgery is the preferred treatment for cancers in the lower third of the esophagus. Depending on the results of clinical tests, a combination of treatments may be recommended. This is particularly true when surgery has been performed but some residual disease is left behind. In these cases, radiation is administered postoperatively.

The radiation therapist must decide if the treatment should be considered *curative* or *palliative*. When radiation therapy is recommended *following* surgery, it is usually administered to control growth and reduce symptoms, and is therefore considered palliative. In these cases there is usually known disease in lymph nodes that surgery can't remove.

Another group of patients is given only radiation therapy. Some patients in this group have only localized disease, and radiation is given to *cure* the cancer without surgery. In other patients the cancer is believed to be inoperable, and therefore the palliative treatment is performed to temporarily stop the growth of the tumor and to relieve symptoms.

Radiation treatments generally extend into normal tissue on either side of the known, or visualized, cancer. This is done because this type of cancer commonly extends beyond the identified area. In addition, radiation is directed to the adjacent lymph nodes in the esophagus.

Treatment is delivered through multiple portals, that is, the front, the back, and each side. On occasion, there is a rotational treatment plan, meaning that the radiation therapy machine rotates around the patient's body. Approximately 5,000 units of radiation are delivered over a six-week period. If there appears to be a good chance for a cure, a higher dose is delivered in seven or eight weeks.

SIDE EFFECTS. Radiation therapy to this area of the body may cause acute symptoms of nausea and vomiting, and irritation of the esophagus makes swallowing painful. Patients with this type of cancer generally have poor nutritional status to begin with because the nature of the illness makes normal eating more difficult. The onset of these side effects begins a cycle that must be managed. It is essential that the radiation therapist direct dietary changes and prescribe medication to reduce side effects.

Pain medication is used for the esophageal irritation. (Xylocaine Viscous, an anesthetic gel, and common over-the-counter pain tablets are used.) Patients generally eat pureed foods, and are also advised to avoid both hot or cold food and liquids. Commercially prepared, nutritionally balanced liquid preparations, available in pharmacies and food markets, are particularly helpful in maintaining sound nutritional status. (I prefer Ensure.) Liquid multivitamin and mineral preparations are also advisable. Nausea and vomiting may be controlled with an antinausea medication such as Compazine. When these strategies are followed, symptoms usually improve and are quite tolerable. In most cases, patients are able to complete radiation therapy.

When an x-ray test called an esophagram is performed halfway through the treatment course, it often reveals significant improvement in the appearance of the esophagus in many cases. When improvement is demonstrated, these patients are then able to increase their intake of solid food.

Delayed complications of radiation therapy may occur many months or years after the treatment is completed. These side effects generally include narrowing, or stricture, of the esophagus or radiation scarring of the adjacent lung. However, since survival rates are generally quite low for this type of cancer, these long-term side effects are seen infrequently.

FOLLOW-UP AND OUTLOOK. Best treatment results are obtained when cancer of the esophagus is found early and has not spread to distant sites. Unfortunately, this cancer often is advanced when detected, in which case the outcome of treatment is poor with either radiation or surgery.

The majority of patients do achieve a relatively good quality of life after radiation treatment, especially when compared to the discomfort associated with radical surgery. When radiation is not successful in achieving a satisfactory result, surgery and chemotherapy are still treatment options. Although chemotherapy has been shown to be useful in shrinking tumors, to date, survival rates have not been improved.

Although we can sometimes control the disease locally, distant metastases are usually responsible for the cause of death. Currently, the only hope for curing this cancer lies in early detection. X-ray esophagrams, endoscopy (examining the esophagus through an inserted tube), and CT scans are used to evaluate the patient's progress.

Head and Neck

Head and neck cancers are a complex group of tumors, and each site of origin has its own individual biological characteristics. Cancers of the *head* include tumors of the tongue, gums, the lining of the mouth, tonsils, sinuses, and lymph tissues above the soft palate. Cancers of the *neck* include those that originate in the vocal cords (larynx) or the adjacent soft tissues (pharynx).

Radiation therapy treatment plans for each of these cancer groups are in principle quite similar. Therefore, all head cancers will be discussed as one group, and all neck cancers as another. Because tumors and normal tissues are located in a small space near one another, vital structures are either included or excluded from the treatment beam. This depends on the particular clinical situation. Extreme precision is necessary in the treatment of these areas, and therefore the radiation therapist, the radiation physicist, and the surgeon work closely together and consult with one another often.

TREATMENT TO THE HEAD. Most tumors of the head are fairly resistant to radiation therapy and therefore require a high total dose of radiation, approximately 6,000 to 7,000 units. Treatments are delivered on a daily basis for a period of six to seven weeks and are usually administered through treatment fields on each side of the head. More complex treatment plans, with radiation delivered through different angles, may be required. The locations for the treatment beams are marked with small temporary tattoos, not visible to others.

Radiation may be the only form of treatment, or it may be administered in an attempt to shrink the tumor before surgery, thereby allowing less radical removal of tissues. Radiation may also be used following surgery if cancer remains. The variation in treatment plans depends on many factors, including the original site of the cancer, its size, and the degree to which it has spread to adjacent tissues and lymph nodes. (The body contains thousands of lymph nodes whose function is to filter elements foreign to the body—common infections and cancer, for example. Because they are widely distributed throughout the body, lymph nodes are often affected as cancer invades tissues around the original site.) The extent of surgery performed is individualized for each patient. As a general rule, patients with cancers of the head have surgery first, which may include removal of adjacent lymph nodes.

Recently, chemotherapy has been shown to be effective in treating these tumors. It may be used before, during, or after radiation treatment. However, if it is administered close to the time radiation is given, many side effects will be aggravated.

SIDE EFFECTS OF TREATMENT TO THE HEAD. The most common symptom resulting from radiation to the head is dry mouth, caused by decreased production of saliva and drying out of the lining of the mouth (mucous membranes). The decreased salivary production can lead to rapid deterioration of the person's dental condition. Patients with preexisting dental problems or poor oral hygiene are advised to see a dentist before radiation treatments begin. A complete dental evaluation prior to radiation is essential to minimize dental side effects. Fluoride treatments, plaque removal, filling cavities, and tooth extractions should all be done prior to treatment. When dental problems exist, infections can result and seriously complicate radiation therapy. Patients who do not need immediate dental work are closely monitored during treatment to insure that decreased saliva does not lead to deterioration of dental health. Routine dental care is recommended, in particular fluoride applications to ensure that dental health status remains satisfactory.

Patients who wear dentures must remove them during treatment, because they interact with the radiation and irritate the mucous membranes in the mouth. Dentures may be replaced after each treatment session. However, the dentures may not fit properly because of the weight loss associated with cancer and the treatment. Once treatment is completed, the dentures may be refitted.

Dry mouth can be minimized by using sugar-free sour candies, sucking on fruit pits, or by using the old remedy of sucking on a button. An artificial saliva product, such as Salivart, is effective, and similar products are constantly being improved. Drugs to stimulate saliva production are being tested and may come on the market shortly. These products act as a lubricant but do not prevent dental problems.

The soreness of the tissues resulting from the radiation may be aggravated by eating and drinking. Taste sensations are also altered during radiation treatment to the head, and thus the enjoyment of eating is markedly reduced. This side effect, resulting from the effects of radiation on the tongue and the decrease of saliva, begins two to three weeks into the course of treatment and lasts throughout the remainder of the treatment course. It may be a month or two before taste sensations return, and the reduced amount of saliva as well as the thickened consistency may persist for months or years after treatment.

Because radiation irritates the tissues lining the mouth, infections may occur that must be treated with antibiotics. If left untreated, local infections may spread to other areas of the body. Oral pain is treated with gels to numb the mouth (I prefer Xylocaine Viscous) or other common pain medications. The skin over the treated area often becomes reddened and dry, and because of the high radiation doses, it may also blister. Skin creams such as Nivea and cortisone ointments are helpful in alleviating these symptoms.

Loss of taste, decreased salivary production, and soreness of the mouth often lead patients to reject food. This sets up a vicious cycle, because the person's nutritional status may have been significantly altered by the presence of the painful tumor, which in turn discouraged eating. Radiation therapy may then aggravate the problem. Family members should attempt to provide nutritional support during this very trying period for the patient. Liquid dietary supplements, available at drug stores and food markets, are valuable because they provide nutritional balance but do not require much effort to ingest. (I prefer a preparation called Ensure.) I also recommend using an ordinary kitchen blender to make drinks and shakes from cooked or raw vegetables. When tolerated, spices can be added to make these drinks appealing. Liquid vitamin and mineral supplements are also advisable if regular food is preferred. Your radiation therapist will monitor your nutritional status and suggest ways to keep calorie intake adequate and balanced.

Radiation therapists monitor progress by physical examination throughout the course of treatment. The size of the treatment field and the angle of the delivery may be modified, depending on the results.

TREATMENT TO THE NECK. Surgery may be the only treatment, and this decision is guided by the location and size of the cancer, as well as its patterns of spread.

Radiation therapy to the *neck* for tumors in the vocal cords and other surrounding structures requires high doses because the tumors may, when large, exhibit some resistance to radiation. Approximately 6,000 to 7,000 units of radiation are usually delivered daily for seven to eight weeks. The treatment beam is directed to each side of the neck, but a more complex approach may be required, depending on the patient's clinical situation.

Radiation may be the only form of treatment and is usually used for early vocal cord cancer. It may also be administered in an attempt to shrink the tumor before surgery, thereby allowing less radical removal of the tissues. Radiation may also be used following surgery if cancer remains. The variation in treatment plans depends on many factors, including the original site of the cancer, its size, and the degree to which it has spread to adjacent tissues and lymph nodes. (The body contains thousands of lymph nodes, whose function it is to filter elements foreign to the body—

common infections and cancer, for example. Because they are widely distributed throughout the body, lymph nodes are often affected as cancer invades tissues around the orginal site.) The extent of surgery performed is individualized for each patient. As a general rule, patients with cancer in the neck have surgery first, which may include removal of adjacent lymph nodes.

SIDE EFFECTS OF TREATMENT TO THE NECK. About two to three weeks into the treatment course, difficulty in swallowing and hoarseness may begin. Some patients are hoarse before therapy begins, particularly those with vocal-cord cancers. Patients also complain of the dryness in the tissues and thickening of the secretions in the throat. They may also experience some pain, particularly when swallowing. This can be partially alleviated by avoiding hot or cold food and liquids. If necessary, the diet can be further modified by following the guidelines discussed in the previous section concerning cancers occurring in the head. However, most patients being treated with radiation for cancers of the neck are able to tolerate foods.

Excess phlegm in the throat can be controlled by using room humidifiers and drinking plenty of fluids. Throughout treatment, everything ingested should be served at room temperature. In addition, alcohol should be avoided and patients must not smoke.

Some reddening of the skin over the area of treatment may occur because of the high dose of radiation necessary to control the cancer. Skin creams such as Nivea and those that contain cortisone, will alleviate discomfort.

A throat infection may develop as well, and may cause cancer-bearing lymph nodes in the neck to become infected, which further aggravates the patient's discomfort. Pain medication and antibiotics are used to treat these symptoms. Patients are also encouraged not to strain their voice if hoarseness is a problem.

These side effects may be troublesome throughout treatment, but they gradually subside once the radiation therapy is complete, and usually disappear in a month or so.

FOLLOW-UP AND OUTLOOK OF TREATMENT TO THE HEAD AND NECK. Results of radiation therapy to the head and neck are evaluated by direct examination of the mouth and throat, either by the surgeon or the radiation therapist. In many instances, it is necessary for an ear, nose, and throat surgeon to insert a tube to look at areas that can't be seen directly by the naked eye, a procedure called endoscopy. It is also essential to have periodic follow-up physical examinations.

CT scans and MRI scans of the head and neck are valuable because they can image tissues not seen by the naked eye or endoscopy. Lymph nodes are also examined with CT and MRI scans (see chapter 9).

If patients have been habitual users of tobacco and alcohol, they are urged to discontinue using them. The combination of the two substances is associated with a high incidence of head and neck cancers.

Hodgkin's Disease

Hodgkin's disease is believed to originate from abnormal cells in the lymph nodes. Human beings have thousands of lymph nodes distributed throughout the body, which filter elements that are foreign to the body—common infections and cancer, for example.

Virtually everyone has had a throat infection that caused lumpy swellings on the sides of the neck. The lymph nodes have filtered the draining infection and have swollen in response to this invasion of a foreign element.

When Hodgkin's disease originates in lymph nodes, these normally small structures grow, but the swellings are often pain-less. More than 80 percent of patients with Hodgkin's disease will have lymph-node swelling in the neck; 50 percent of patients will have lymph-node swelling in the middle portion of the chest, known as the mediastinum.

Hodgkin's disease has a marked tendency to affect lymph nodes in adjacent body tissues. For example, if lymph nodes in the upper neck are involved first, the next affected areas will likely be the lower neck and the upper shoulder area, the chest,

and the underarm region. This biological fact is of great importance when planning radiation treatment.

In most patients, Hodgkin's disease does not cause symptoms other than the swelling of the lymph nodes. However,
approximately one third of Hodgkin's patients have fevers,
weight loss, and anemia. The presence of these symptoms usually
indicates a more serious stage of the disease.

TREATMENT. Following the diagnosis, by means of a biopsy of a
lymph node, the radiation therapist plans treatment directed to
the involved lymph nodes and those that are adjacent but not
yet known to be affected. Therefore, radiation treatments for
known Hodgkin's disease in the neck and chest would include all
the lymph nodes in the neck and chest as well as adjacent nodes
in the upper shoulder and underarm region. In these situations,
the lymph nodes in the abdomen may be similarly treated, even
if there is no conclusive evidence that the disease has invaded
these structures, because the path of the disease may extend
downward through the body.

Radiation therapy to the lymph nodes in the chest is administered in one stage, usually lasting four to five weeks, in which a
total of about 4,000 units of radiation may be delivered.
Following an interruption in treatments to allow the body to
recover, a second course of radiation therapy to the abdomen
may begin, depending on the clinical situation.

Some patients with Hodgkin's disease require a combination of treatments. For example, some patients have chest and
abdominal lymph-node disease simultaneously, discovered by
CT scans of the chest, abdomen, and pelvis and also by lymphangiograms (see chapter 9). This group of patients will be given
a combination of chemotherapy and radiation treatment. A
splenectomy (removal of the spleen) may be performed if this
organ is involved. Patients whose disease is in both the chest and
abdomen are considered to have advanced-stage Hodgkin's disease. The chemotherapy treatment usually consists of four chemical agents with the acronym MOPP. Chemotherapy may be the
only treatment given, and radiation therapy is reserved to later
treat persistent disease.

Radiation treatments are performed through the front and
the back of the patient. Vital structures that do not require

radiation must be blocked; great care is taken to design heart, thyroid gland, and lung blocks so as to "shape" the treatment field in the chest. Kidney and liver blocks are used to shape the treatment field in the abdominal area. The resulting shaped radiation field on the chest and neck is commonly known as *mantle* treatment.

SIDE EFFECTS. The acute side effects of radiation therapy to the chest and neck include some hair loss on the back of the head, occasionally nausea, sore throat, some dryness in the mouth, and mild reddening of the skin over the areas being treated. Dryness of the mouth can be alleviated by drinking plenty of fluids and by sucking on sour, hard candy. Skin irritation can be relieved with a soothing skin cream. (I prefer Nivea.) Nausea can be treated with Compazine.

Nausea and occasional diarrhea occur when treatment is directed to the abdomen. These symptoms can be treated with Compazine and Lomotil respectively.

With the exception of the hair loss, these symptoms are easily controlled with medication. They are *acute* in that they appear during the treatment course but promptly disappear when radiation therapy is completed. These acute symptoms are generally more of an annoyance than a serious problem.

Throughout the course of treatment, the patient's blood count is carefully monitored because the large radiation fields, which include the bones, affect the bone marrow. This can result in a lowering of the white blood-cell count, which then compromises the body's ability to fight infection. Platelets, another blood cell manufactured in the marrow, may also be reduced, causing small hemorrhages to occur. Treatment may need to be interrupted until the blood count returns to normal. Recently, drugs have been developed that stimulate formation of blood cells. However, they have side effects of their own.

Some chronic complications (as opposed to those symptoms that are acute and disappear) may result from this extensive radiation treatment to the lymph nodes. For example, thyroid dysfunction is possible; however, it can be treated should it occur. Persistent dryness of the mouth may result in an increase of dental problems that require regular follow-up care. On occasion, pneumonia may develop as a result of radiation to the lung, and cortisone medication may be required to treat the condition. Similarly, there is a possibility that a radiation-induced heart condition may occur, usually involving fluid formation in the lining of the tissues around the heart. Medication or surgery may be necessary to correct this condition. Although careful blocking of tissues during treatment reduces the incidence of these complications, they are not entirely avoidable.

The most serious long-term side effect of treatment of Hodgkin's disease is the possible development of other cancers years later. This is most often seen in those patients who have received chemotherapy together with radiation, because it is generally accepted that aggressive chemotherapy and radiation treatment may depress the immune system, thus allowing for the later development of other cancers. For example, there is a greater incidence of secondary leukemia and non-Hodgkin's lymphoma among these patients than there is in the normal population. However, the good news is that with these aggressive treatments, many more patients with Hodgkin's disease are currently being *cured* than in the past. In fact, much of the improvement in cancer survival statistics is related to the increase in the cure rate for Hodgkin's disease.

Most male patients and half of the female patients become sterile as a result of the *combination* of radiation and chemotherapy. An operation known as oophoropexy, which moves a woman's ovaries out of the path of the radiation beam, may be an option, depending on the individual's clinical situation. Some male patients may consider placing sperm in a sperm bank before undergoing radiation treatment or chemotherapy. However, for reasons not well understood, some patients (both men and women) with advanced Hodgkin's disease may already be infertile as a result of their disease. Fertility is a complex issue for patients with Hodgkin's disease, and I urge my patients to seek fertility counseling before starting treatment.

FOLLOW-UP AND OUTLOOK. Hodgkin's disease may affect sites other than the lymph nodes. These sites are also treated with combinations of radiation therapy and chemotherapy, depending on the size and location of the cancer.

Follow-up evaluation of the treatment results includes blood tests and physical examination of the lymph nodes and organs such as the spleen and liver. CT scans of the chest and abdomen are particularly useful when evaluating the size of chest and abdominal lymph nodes (see chapter 9).

Radiation therapy and multiagent chemotherapy and aggressive combinations of both treatment methods have resulted in significant improvements in the five-year survival rate for Hodgkin's disease. Over the past 40 years, the survival rate has more than doubled, and Hodgkin's disease is now considered *curable* in early stages as well as when it is moderately advanced.

Lung

Lung cancers most often develop in the cells that line the bronchial tubes. Because lung cancer often initially causes few symptoms, it is frequently first diagnosed incidentally on a routine chest x-ray. However, some patients may complain of a chronic cough or unexplained weight loss; some develop a pneumonia that does not heal in spite of treatment.

A biopsy is necessary to make a definitive diagnosis, and it can be accomplished in one of two ways. In the first, a flexible tube is passed into the bronchial tree of the lung, enabling the physician to obtain a small piece of tissue to examine, or to obtain cells that have sloughed from the tumor into the bronchial tree. In the second, a fine needle is passed through the chest under local anesthesia to the suspected tumor with the guidance of a CT scan (see chapter 9). A CT scan will also be performed to see if the tumor has spread beyond the lung into the adjacent lymph nodes in the center of the chest. (Human beings have thousands of lymph nodes, which act as filters for elements that are foreign to the body—infections and cancer, for example. Because lymph nodes are so widely distributed, they are often affected when cancer begins to spread from its original site to adjacent tissues.) The abdomen and brain may also be scanned to determine if additional organs are involved. This evaluation is necessary before physicians can design a treatment plan that is appropriate for the particular stage of the disease.

It is rare for patients with lung cancer to feel very ill from the cancer itself at the time they begin radiation therapy. The exception occurs when the cancer has obstructed the bronchial tubes or caused extensive pressure on the major blood vessels.

Difficulties arise when the tumor cells compete with the normal cells for nutrition, so that the patients' fatigue and illness are caused by poor nutritional status and general malaise. In many cases, the tumor is significantly arrested and patients note a marked improvement in the way they feel within a month or two following completion of treatment. The major problems that arise with lung cancer are those that occur when the cancer spreads to distant sites. In these cases the symptoms may be very debilitating.

TREATMENT. At the present time, there is considerable controversy surrounding the treatment of lung cancer because of the increased use of chemotherapy. The treatment approaches described here are those that I and many radiation therapists currently favor. However, these treatments may change in the future as more clinical data is acquired. The discussions about the best treatments are legitimate and important, and patients today have options that were at one time not available. Therefore, patients are encouraged to seek additional opinions about any treatments presented here.

If the cancer is restricted to the lung, then surgery is performed, generally entailing removal of all (pneumonectomy) or part (lobectomy) of a lung. A person's age and overall physical condition are factors considered when determining if surgery will be performed.

If the patient is considered to be at high risk for surgery because of medical problems (usually chronic lung disease) and the cancer is in the early stage, radiation therapy is administered to attempt to cure the disease.

Patients who are able to tolerate surgery are referred for radiation therapy following surgery if lymph nodes are also discovered to contain cancer.

When, prior to surgery, a CT scan has revealed that lymph- node involvement is extensive or that the tumor itself is very extensive, the patient is referred to radiation therapy *only*.

The purpose of the radiation treatment is to arrest the cancer, even though at that stage the disease is not considered curable.

In about 20 percent of lung-cancer patients, the type of cancer cell present is unusually aggressive. (This is known as *small cell* or *oat cell* carcinoma.) In these cases, the brain, liver, and bone are evaluated because the tumor is so aggressive that cancer frequently coexists there or rapidly spreads to these sites. Surgery is not performed in these cases, and chemotherapy is the primary mode of treatment. Radiation therapy then supplements the chemotherapy if necessary.

Most patients referred for radiation treatment usually have a six- or seven-week course of treatment. When radiation is the primary treatment, approximately 6,000 units of radiation may be delivered. Less radiation may be used in patients who have had surgery or chemotherapy.

Sometimes the cancer may cause special problems. These involve extensive bleeding from the lung or rapid onset of shortness of breath because the large blood vessels or the bronchi are obstructed. In these cases, the daily and total dosage of radiation will be altered. The daily treatments may then be delivered in high doses in the often successful attempt to reduce these acute symptoms.

Radiation is delivered daily to the front and back of the chest or at different angles, with the portal arrangement tailored to the particular clinical picture. Treatment includes the lung tumor itself, if it has not been surgically removed, plus all the nearby lymph nodes.

Radiation treatment can control the local primary tumor much of the time. However, by the time many lung cancers are diagnosed, they are already in an advanced stage and the cancer has spread to other parts of the body. Some of these metastases (areas of the spreading disease) may be clinically detectable at the time of the diagnostic work-up. Unfortunately, many are not detected until after the primary cancer has been treated.

Chemotherapy for lung cancer is often administered prior to surgery (neoadjuvant therapy) or postoperatively. Survival among patients who are treated with surgery, radiation, and multidose chemotherapy is significantly higher than for those patients who have only surgery. When the patient is not a good candidate for surgery, I prefer to administer radiation *prior* to chemotherapy. When administered first, chemotherapy significantly lowers the patient's ability to tolerate the radiation therapy. (There is considerable controversy in the medical literature over the sequence of these treatments.)

The total radiation dose and the daily dose may be modified if the patient is also receiving chemotherapy, because the tissues may be less able to tolerate radiation while chemotherapy is being administered.

Multiagent chemotherapy is the treatment of choice for the *small cell* cancers mentioned earlier. In this type of cancer, tumor size will rapidly decrease in about 70 percent of patients. The tumor can then be treated with radiation if chemotherapy has resulted in only a partial response (see chapter 7).

SIDE EFFECTS. The side effects of radiation therapy to the chest are generally moderate, and most patients are able to pursue their normal lifestyles. However, many patients complain of fatigue, which generally disappears approximately one month after radiation therapy is completed. Although patients are encouraged to work and carry out their normal daily activities, the fatigue can sometimes make doing so too difficult. Underlying and preexisting physical conditions and, of course, mental attitude will influence a person's lifestyle.

Side effects begin approximately two to three weeks after treatment has started. The primary side effect is moderate irritation of the esophagus, the swallowing tube. However, there is wide variation in the severity of this symptom. Some people may report very little difficulty; others may find this symptom quite annoying.

Liquid antacids help to soothe the esophagus, and I advise patients to avoid either very hot or very cold foods and liquids. I also recommend that patients avoid spicy foods because they may cause further irritation. Chewing foods well before swallowing is also advantageous. Some, but by no means all, patients complain of moderate nausea. The drug Compazine usually controls this symptom. On occasion, a radiation-induced cough appears. This is actually a mild bronchitis brought on by the radiation. Various cough remedies relieve this problem, and it is never a serious side effect. These side effects generally disappear a week or two after completion of treatment.

Because of their weakened state, some patients may develop an infection, and antibiotics are needed to control it. More rarely, a patient may develop mild radiation-induced pneumonia one to two months after radiation treatment is finished. Antibiotics and cortisone may be used to treat this condition.

FOLLOW-UP AND OUTLOOK. Follow-up treatment for lung cancer includes regular chest x-rays to detect recurrent disease and CT scans of the chest and abdomen. Lung cancer most commonly spreads to the bone, liver, and brain. If symptoms appear, diagnostic tests generally ordered include a CT scan of the brain, a CT scan of the abdomen to evaluate the liver, and a nuclear bone scan if bone symptoms are present (see chapter 9). Blood tests for liver function that can reveal signs of early liver disease are also performed.

Although the cure rate for lung cancer is low because of the high incidence of distant metastases present at the time it is detected, I have had personal experience with cures. Therefore, I recommend that an aggressive treatment program be instituted to achieve the maximum benefits.

Multiple Myeloma

Multiple myeloma originates in plasma cells. When plasma cells multiply in an uncontrolled fashion, they cause abnormalities, generally in the skeleton. When the condition affects one bone, it is called solitary myeloma; when it affects many bones, it is considered multiple myeloma. Other sites in the body, such as the nasal passages, the sinuses, the lungs, the lymph nodes, the kidneys, and bone marrow can be affected, but this occurs less frequently. Myeloma causes pain in the affected bones, and the patient has an increased susceptibility to infection. Multiple myeloma is often associated with remissions (improvements) and exacerbations (flare-ups). The remissions can occur spontaneously or as a result of treatment.

TREATMENT. Although there is no known cure, chemotherapy is the primary treatment for controlling myeloma. Radiation therapy is used to control bone pain and to shrink masses that may be disfiguring. It is also performed to relieve compression of the spinal cord and nerve roots if the disease has spread to this area of the body.

Most patients receiving radiation therapy for multiple myeloma report prompt relief of the bone pain, and the masses usually shrink rapidly. If treatment has been initiated early, when myeloma affects the spinal cord and nerves, normal nerve function can be restored.

Doses of 2,000 to 4,000 units of radiation may be administered over a two- to four-week period, usually without significant side effects. There is a wide variation of response to the treatment. Some patients obtain prompt relief of symptoms with 2,000 units; others need the higher dose of 4,000 units for the same symptom relief.

SIDE EFFECTS. When treatment is delivered to the long bones of the arms and legs, no side effects are expected. However, when radiation treatments are directed to the spine, the patient may experience symptoms if enough radiation reaches adjacent soft tissues. For example, treatments to the neck might cause a sore throat; treatments to the lower spine might cause nausea. These symptoms can be alleviated with medication and dietary modifications (see chapters 2 and 3).

FOLLOW-UP AND OUTLOOK. It is unusual, but not impossible, for the disease to recur in the treated area. Those patients who have initially received a lower dose of radiation may need to return for additional treatment to the same areas. However, multiple myeloma is usually characterized by new growths, which, over time, appear in other parts of the body. For this reason, many patients are seen over a period of months for additional treatment to different bones in the body.

Chemotherapy may eliminate bone pain and temporarily halt the progression of the disease. Unfortunately, chemotherapy often depresses the bone marrow's ability to manufacture new platelets, causing a tendency to bleed, and red and white blood cells, which lowers the body's ability to fight infection. Bacterial infections may result from weakened immunity. In addition, long-term consequences of this treatment may include acute leukemia.

Both radiation and chemotherapy are quite effective in temporarily arresting multiple myeloma, and about 90 percent of patients will obtain good pain relief. Those patients whose disease progresses slowly may live for many years. However, in some patients multiple myeloma is much more aggressive and only short-term survival is possible. Specialized blood and urine tests help determine the aggressiveness of the disease in individual patients.

X-rays and CT scans of the affected bones and other areas of the body are commonly used to evaluate the results of treatment and detect new disease.

Non-Hodgkin's Lymphoma

Non-Hodgkin's lymphomas are a group of diseases in which abnormal cells develop in lymph nodes; the disease may then spread to other sites throughout the body. Human beings have thousands of lymph nodes distributed throughout the body. They trap elements foreign to the body—infections and cancer, for example. This type of lymphoma is different from Hodgkin's disease in the way in which it spreads. Rather than moving to adjacent lymph-node groups in a step-by-step progression, its spread is much less predictable. Non-Hodgkin's lymphomas also tend to affect an older population than Hodgkin's disease, which usually affects younger people. Non-Hodgkin's lymphomas also frequently involve the bone marrow.

The rise in the number of AIDS patients has resulted in increasing cases of non-Hodgkin's lymphoma. This is probably the result of immunosuppression, or the weakening of the body's own defenses.

Unfortunately, many patients with non-Hodgkin's lymphomas already have advanced disease by the time they are diagnosed. Patients fall into two major groups. The first has a nonaggressive type of cancer cell, and these patients may survive for many years. The second group of patients has a very aggressive type of cancer, and survival time is shorter. In either group, the disease may affect one or many areas of the body. This disease is often associated with remissions (improvements) and exacerbations (flare-ups). The remissions can occur spontaneously or as a result of the treatment

TREATMENT. Radiation therapy is given to patients with localized lymph-node disease and may be the only treatment necessary. Those patients with disease (either the aggressive or non-aggressive type) in many lymph nodes throughout the body may need radiation therapy following chemotherapy if the cancer remains extensive.

It is common for this disease to be generalized, that is, it affects many organs and body systems. In these cases, chemotherapy is particularly useful because it reaches all parts of the body.

Radiation therapy is often successful in treating local disease in the advanced stages of non-Hodgkin's lymphoma when chemotherapy is no longer effective. Radiation shrinks the tumors, alleviates pain, and reduces swelling in the tissues. It is particularly beneficial for treating large lymph nodes, the nasal passages, the bones, the spine, the intestinal tract, and the brain. A total of 4,000 to 5,000 units of radiation may be delivered in daily treatments over a four- to five-week period.

Surgery (biopsy) is used to make a tissue diagnosis, to identify the cell type as aggressive or nonaggressive, and then to determine how extensive the disease is (the stage). Occasionally, surgery is performed to remove a tumor, particularly from the intestinal tract.

SIDE EFFECTS. Expected side effects of radiation therapy depend on the part of the body being treated. For example, dryness of the mouth and painful swallowing are common when treatment is delivered to the head and neck. Nausea and vomiting are likely to occur when treatment is directed to the abdomen. Appropriate medications and dietary modifications will help alleviate these symptoms (see chapters 2 and 3). When large areas of the chest or abdomen are treated, the considerable irradiation of the bone marrow may lead to a lowered white and red blood-cell count and platelets. These symptoms may be aggravated if chemotherapy is given either simultaneously or immediately before the radiation treatment (see chapter 7).

FOLLOW-UP AND OUTLOOK. Combined chemotherapy and radiation have resulted in significantly increased five-year survival rates. However, it is discouraging to note that incidence of this disease is increasing.

To date, radiation and chemotherapy can offer patients relief of symptoms and excellent control of the disease. However, the disease will ultimately overwhelm the body. Because so much progress has been made in arresting this disease during the past several decades, it is hoped that as new treatments are discovered, survival rates will increase.

CT scans and MRI scans are used to evaluate the results of treatment. Nuclear scans are also used if bones are involved in the disease (see chapter 9).

Pancreas

The pancreas, a gland located in the abdomen near the stomach, is responsible for manufacturing digestive juices. In its early stages, pancreatic cancer is usually *silent*, in that it doesn't cause symptoms. When symptoms appear, they generally include gradual weight loss, pain, and, depending on location, jaundice (yellowing of the skin).

The cancer is often best detected with a CT scan (see chapter 9) followed by a biopsy, which is necessary for a definitive diagnosis. Chemicals known as *tumor markers*, which indicate the presence of cancer, have recently been discovered in the blood. The specific chemical that is frequently increased in this cancer is the carcinoembryonic antigen (CEA). Detecting this chemical is useful in establishing the diagnosis and in evaluating the results of treatment.

TREATMENT. Surgery is frequently performed for this cancer, but unfortunately, by the time it is discovered, the disease is often found to be incurable. Recent clinical studies have found that aggressive radiation therapy combined with chemotherapy may be as effective as surgery in controlling this disease. When radiation treatment and chemotherapy are used together, with or without surgery, five-year survival statistics have been shown to improve.

Patients who are not considered likely to be cured will sometimes have some tumor tissue removed in order relieve obstruction of the bile ducts. (When present, this obstruction may cause jaundice.)

Approximately 4,000 units of radiation are delivered to the pancreas through the front and the back of the body. The treatment course may be continuous for four to five weeks, or it may be divided into two 2,000-unit courses with an interval of several weeks between each course.

The kidneys, portions of the liver, the intestines, and the stomach are shielded from unnecessary levels of radiation. The radiation treatment field includes the adjacent lymph nodes. (Human beings have thousands of lymph nodes, which act as filters for elements foreign to the body—infection and cancer, for example. Because they are so widely distributed throughout the body, lymph nodes often are affected when cancer begins to spread from its original site to adjacent tissues.)

SIDE EFFECTS. Many people undergo radiation treatment to the pancreas and experience only moderate side effects. Some may experience nausea and heartburn, but these side effects are easily controlled with medication (Compazine and antacids). Most patients use a trial-and-error method to determine which foods must be avoided. Generally speaking, low-fat, bland foods are best (see chapter 3). Commercial liquid dietary preparations are often excellent food sources because they contain required calories and include vitamins and minerals but require little effort to ingest. These products are available in pharmacies and food markets (I prefer Ensure). Liquid vitamin and mineral supplements are advisable for people who prefer regular foods but are unable to consume enough to provide adequate nutrition.

Nausea and vomiting are common side effects of chemotherapy, and when radiation is given simultaneously, symptoms may be aggravated. Occasional pain resulting from radiation can be treated with over-the-counter medication. Severe pain is often caused by the disease and may require narcotics. (If patients have had extensive surgery, a gastroen-terologist will prescribe pancreatic juice preparations, which take the place of the digestive juices ordinarily produced by the pancreas and necessary for normal absorption of nutrients.)

FOLLOW-UP AND OUTLOOK. Treatment results can best be eval-uated by performing a CT scan of the abdomen. A CT scan will also help determine if there has been regrowth of the cancer and whether it has spread to neighboring organs. CEA levels are also taken to measure tumor activity. A drop in CEA values is a good sign; rising values indicate that the cancer is regrowing.

When used in combination, radiation therapy and chemo-therapy often reverse the jaundice, pain, and weight loss caused by the cancer. However, by the time most patients are diagnosed, pancreatic cancer is usually in an advanced stage, so that sur-vival rates are low. Cures do occur, so when indicated, treatment should be aggressive.

Prostate

The prostate gland, an organ of the male reproductive system, lies at the outlet of the urinary bladder and in front of the rec-tum. The development of cancer in this gland is quite common in males, second only to cancer in the lung. It is also an unpre-dictable form of cancer. In some patients it will progress very rapidly; in others it develops slowly over a period of many years. For this reason, treatment is determined on a case-by-case basis, and generalities aren't easily made.

This type of cancer is often detected incidentally during surgery for benign (nonmalignant) enlargement of the prostate (benign prostatic hypertrophy), a common condition among older men. In a way, this is a fortunate event, because many of these cancers are small and confined to the prostate itself. In other words, the cancer is found before it has spread to other organs.

Prostate cancer may also be discovered during rectal examinations performed as part of a routine physical. The physi-cian will detect a hard nodule when the prostate is manually examined, and a biopsy is performed to confirm or exclude the diagnosis of cancer. This group of patients may have either early or more advanced disease.

Another group of patients may seek medical help because of bone pain. On investigation it is learned that the cancer has spread to the bone from an unsuspected prostate cancer. These patients are in the most advanced stage of the disease, and overall survival rates are lower.

Once cancer of the prostate has been confirmed, further testing is done to determine if the cancer has spread beyond the prostate into the surrounding tissues and lymph nodes. Abdominal and pelvic CT scans are used for the additional evaluations (see chapter 9). In this particular situation, a CT scan is only moderately sensitive, and therefore other tests are performed in order to get as complete an evaluation as possible. Ultrasound examinations of the prostate are now being used to help increase the accuracy of the biopsy.

Highly specialized blood tests can assist in evaluating for the spread of cancer outside the prostate. Elevated levels of a chemical, prostatic specific antigen (PSA), usually indicate that cancer is present and may have spread beyond the gland itself. PSA levels can also be elevated in *nonmalignant disease* if the prostate gland is large. (The PSA is currently used as a screening test to detect this cancer.) Later, after surgery or radiation treatment, the PSA test is used to determine the effectiveness of the treatment. The values of the PSA should fall; a rise indicates tumor activity and may require diagnostic work-up.

A nuclear bone scan (see chapter 9) is performed to determine if the cancer has spread to the bones. Surgery may also be performed to determine if cancer is present in the pelvic lymph nodes. These tests and procedures, performed prior to treatment, help clarify the stage of the cancer.

TREATMENT. When preliminary testing suggests that the cancer is localized, that is, confined to the prostate, the patient may undergo surgery, a course of radiation therapy, or both. More than in many other cancers it is the patient's personal choice, and is a matter of weighing the pros and cons. The discovery of cancer in lymph nodes adjacent to the prostate, through surgery or x-ray testing, will influence treatment decisions. (The human body has thousands of lymph nodes, which filter elements that are foreign to the body—infections and cancer, for example. Because lymph nodes are so widely distributed throughout the body, they are often affected when cancer begins to spread from its original site to adjacent tissues.)

The treatments described here may change in the future as more clinical data is acquired. The discussions about the best treatments are legitimate and important, and patients today have options that were at one time not available. Therefore, patients are encouraged to seek additional opinions about any treatment presented.

Surgery involves not only removal of the prostate but much of the surrounding tissues and lymph nodes, a procedure known as a radical prostatectomy. It is major surgery and may lead to impotence and urinary incontinence (loss of voluntary control of urine) in spite of new surgical procedures to prevent damage to the nerve pathways to the prostate.

When cancer is confined to the prostate, surgery is associated with a high cure rate, and many patients choose this option. However, such factors as age and the patient's overall health are considered in the surgical decision, because the surgery is very extensive.

Because many patients who have prostate cancer are in an older age group, normal life expectancy may be limited, and these patients may also have medical conditions that do not allow surgery to be performed. Therefore, many patients in this older age group choose to undergo high-dose radiation therapy instead of surgery because the survival rates are also quite good. Potency is preserved in many cases, and there is minimal incidence of incontinence. In my experience, men in their 60s and older choose to undergo radiation therapy only. There are some patients in an older age group whose disease is early and not aggressive. These cancers can be monitored without administering treatment.

Patients considered good candidates for surgery may also undergo radiation therapy following removal of the prostate gland in order to treat lymph nodes that are found to contain cancer. The removal of some cancerous lymph nodes generally indicates that cancer exists in others.

When radiation is the only treatment, it is generally given daily for approximately seven or eight weeks. A total of 6,000 to 7,000 units of radiation may be delivered to the prostate gland, and a lesser amount (approximately 4,500 to 5,000 units) to the pelvic nodes. Most radiation centers treat pelvic lymph nodes, because it has been determined that a considerable number of patients thought to have an early-stage cancer limited to the prostate in fact have lymph-node involvement. Treatments are generally administered to the front, back, and sides. Rotational treatments, meaning that the machine moves around the patient, are also commonly used. A combination of these methods is also used, an approach I favor.

Patients who have undergone radical prostatectomy and who are referred for radiation therapy to lymph nodes that contain cancer will receive smaller treatment fields and reduced doses of radiation. There are still considerable differences of opinion about which of these patients need lymph-node treatment and about the dosage level necessary.

The radiation treatment described above is *external* radiation, in that it is delivered by machines outside of the body. However, an alternative to this treatment is the use of radioactive sources implanted, that is, placed surgically in the prostate. These radioactive seeds deliver many thousands of units of radiation to the prostate. The implanted seed treats only the prostate gland and does not affect surrounding lymph nodes. Generally, only those patients who have no known lymph-node involvement are considered candidates for this treatment. The radioactivity gradually diminishes over time, eventually approaching zero.

When it has been documented that the prostate cancer has metastasized, usually to the bone, hormonal therapy is instituted. The male hormone, testosterone, is known to stimulate prostate cancer growth, and removing testicular tissue (orchiectomy) decreases production of this hormone. In past years, estrogen, the female hormone, was used to suppress testosterone. Currently, the medication flutamide (Eulexin), in combination with a hormone, has been shown to depress tumor cell activity by blocking the effect of testosterone on the cancer cells. In addition to being very expensive, the drug also leads to problematic weight gain.

If metastases occur, they usually appear in the skeleton, although most organs can be affected (see chapter 6). The spread of metastatic prostate cancer to the spine and the spinal cord may constitute a radiation therapy emergency, in that it must be done immediately to prevent permanent neurological damage.

External beam radiation therapy (See chapter 6) is very effective in reducing bone pain from prostate cancer. Recently, the addition of an isotope (a radioactive substance) called Strontium-89, given by injection into the blood stream, has been found to be very valuable in treating bone pain and prostate cancer. This treatment is usually used when multiple bones are affected by the disease. Pain relief usually begins 10 to 20 days after therapy is started, with maximum relief occurring in about six weeks. There may be a temporary increase in bone pain about one week into treatment, followed by decreased pain in about 80 percent of patients.

The isotope goes specifically to the diseased areas and spares the normal bones of unnecessary levels of radiation. Within one week of administration, 90 percent of the isotope is excreted from the body. The pain relief benefit of this treatment generally lasts between 7 and 12 months. It may also be used in conjunction with external beam radiation therapy to enhance pain relief. Patients will have blood counts checked during and after treatment because the platelet count occasionally decreases.

Average survival is unfortunately only one to three years after the discovery of metastatic prostate cancer. Patients who die of metastatic prostate cancer often had their original prostate cancer cured.

SIDE EFFECTS. Because high doses of radiation are required, most patients will experience side effects. The radiation to the intestines will cause cramping and diarrhea, beginning by the end of the second week or early in the third week of treatment. Medications such as Lomotil, paregoric, or Imodium A-D will usually reduce these intestinal symptoms when combined with dietary modification. The diet should be low in fat, and fried foods and raw fruits and vegetables should also be avoided. All food and liquids should be caffeine-free (see chapter 3). The medication and diet modification must be continued throughout the course of the treatment or symptoms will return.

The bladder is also affected by the high doses of radiation. Urinary urgency and frequency, beginning in the third or fourth week of treatment, are the result of the irritation to the bladder.

Fortunately, medications are available to soothe the bladder (I prefer Pyridium). Sitting in a warm bath twice a day, particularly before going to bed at night, is quite helpful.

Slight blistering and reddening in the rectal area and between the folds of the buttocks are quite common, and generally begin around the fourth or fifth week of treatment. Hydrocortisone cream and Anusol-HC suppositories relieve these symptoms.

The symptoms experienced are predictable, meaning that most people undergoing high-dose radiation therapy for this length of time report similar side effects. I urge you to discuss the symptoms with your radiation therapist as soon as you begin to notice them. There is no need to suffer in silence, because over the years we have found that various medications and dietary modifications can greatly relieve these unpleasant side effects of treatment.

Fortunately, these symptoms disappear within two or three weeks after radiation therapy is complete. It is an unusual patient whose symptoms persist for longer periods. Patients with such underlying medical conditions as ileitis and colitis will be more prone to intestinal side effects, both in the acute stage and over the long term. It is advantageous to stay on the medications and maintain the dietary modifications for at least a week after radiation therapy is complete, because the symptoms diminish gradually rather than disappearing all at once.

About 10 percent of patients will experience transient episodes of bleeding from the rectum or the bladder in the two years following treatment. It is unclear why some patients' intestinal tracts and bladders are more prone to the *delayed* effects of radiation than others. Bleeding may be slight to moderate and usually subsides spontaneously; however, on occasion cauterization may be needed to stop the episodes of bleeding.

Impotency, if it is to occur at all as a result of radiation treatment, usually begins within six months after treatment has been completed. Statistically, we know that approximately 15 percent to 30 percent of previously potent patients develop impotency within two years following completion of treatment. Recently, the new nerve-sparing surgical techniques that attempt to preserve potency and decrease the incidence of incontinence have been favorable factors that allow some men to choose surgery over radiation.

As with all types of cancer, there are normal emotional reactions to having the disease and dealing with the side effects of treatment (see chapters 2 and 4). Both patients and family members may need help to cope with the inevitable difficulties that arise.

FOLLOW-UP AND OUTLOOK. It is mandatory that you see your urologist frequently following completion of treatment. Routine nuclear bone scans are performed for follow-up, because it is quite common for prostate cancer to spread to the bone. This may be *silent* at first, meaning that no symptoms are present. More often, patients complain of bone or muscle pains. The bone scan can detect the first signs of cancer in the bones, thereby allowing treatment to begin early. Together with appropriate x-rays, the bone scan differentiates between the pain of arthritis, for example, and that of cancer. Chest x-rays are also routinely performed, because prostate cancer may spread to the lungs. CT scans are ordered to monitor lymph nodes. Patients will undergo periodic rectal examinations, particularly those whose prostates were not removed. They will also have blood studies (PSA) as described above. PSA levels should fall; a rise indicates tumor activity.

Because the incidence of prostate cancer increases dramatically with age, it is important for men 50 and older to undergo a prostate examination—including a rectal examination and a PSA blood test—at least once a year.

Skin

There are many types of skin cancer, the most common of all cancers. Those usually treated with radiation therapy are basal cell cancer, squamous cell cancer, and Kaposi's sarcoma, often, but not always, associated with AIDS. Melanoma, a very serious form of skin cancer, is usually not effectively treated with radiation unless it has spread to the bones. Squamous cell and basal cell cancer are the most common skin cancers treated with radiation.

TREATMENT. At one time, radiation therapy, surgery, or a combination of both, were the usual methods of treating skin cancer. However, we now have new treatment techniques available, including electrodesiccation, cryosurgery, laser surgery, Mohs micrographic surgery, and topical (local) chemotherapy. Nowadays, those patients referred for radiation therapy for basal or squamous cell cancers are generally elderly persons who may not be willing or able to undergo surgery. Others are treated with radiation therapy if residual disease is present following surgery. I am currently treating fewer skin cancers because of the alternative therapies now available.

When tumors are large, radiation therapy is advantageous because it eliminates the need for complicated surgical procedures, which may require skin grafts. For this reason, it is often the preferred treatment for cancers occurring on the nose, ear, or near the eyes.

Following a diagnostic biopsy, treatment for basal cell cancers is delivered with either superficial radiation therapy machines or with electron beam (see chapter 1). This particular energy of radiation therapy predominantly affects the skin and minimizes radiation to underlying tissues. Doses of 4,000 to 5,000 units of radiation may be delivered over a three- to four-week period of daily treatments. However, doses and treatment schedules vary widely.

The skin being treated eventually reddens, a desirable sign because it indicates that sufficient radiation is reaching the cancer. Some patients have an ulceration of the skin that is caused by the cancer or is the result of the biopsy. A scab, known as an eschar, is often present over the area of ulceration. When treatment is complete, the scab will gradually be shed as the underlying skin heals after the cancer is destroyed.

There are similar treatment plans for squamous cell cancer, although a higher total dose of radiation may be necessary. If the basal or squamous cancer is very extensive, and particularly if it extends to underlying bone or cartilage, a modification of the daily and total dose may be indicated to reduce radiation-therapy complications. Treatments are individualized, and your radiation therapist will make recommendations based on his or her experience and judgment.

Kaposi's sarcoma was a rare cancer. For many years, I treated only an occasional patient for this condition. However, there has been a dramatic increase in cases of this particular cancer because of the immunosuppression that is part of AIDS. The condition is characterized by raised purplish lesions of the skin, the lining of the mouth, lymph nodes, gastrointestinal tract, liver, and spleen.

There are few cures of Kaposi's sarcoma when associated with AIDS, and the main objective of treatment is to improve appearance. Electron-beam therapy is generally used, and the course of radiation is usually short, consisting of 2,000 units of radiation administered in five to six treatments.

SIDE EFFECTS. Patients are often surprised when a skin reaction does not appear immediately. However, it is only toward the end of treatment, usually after three to four weeks, that the skin shows a sunburnlike reaction, which is technically known as a erythema. It persists for many weeks following the end of therapy. Appropriate skin creams (vitamin A and E creams and Nivea) alleviate discomfort.

A raw wound (ulcer) often caused by the cancer will heal within several weeks following radiation treatment, and careful follow-up with the radiation therapist and a dermatologist is necessary. As a rule, the skin is healed two months after treatment is completed.

The reactions experienced by fair-skinned people will be more intense than those experienced by darker-skinned people. Following completion of radiation therapy, a gradual darkening of the skin may occur with some scaling and itching. Ointments and creams are applied as needed according to each individual's reaction. For the most part, the skin returns to its normal appearance in three to six months following completion of radiation therapy. There is, however, great variation among individuals.

FOLLOW-UP AND OUTLOOK. Cure rates for primary basal cell cancer treated with radiation are quite high. However, skin cancer patients must see their dermatologists on a routine basis. This is absolutely necessary, because new tumors arise within a year in 20 to 30 percent of cases. Patients are also advised to avoid excessive exposure to the sun, and they should regularly apply a strong sun block. In some cases, complications may arise. Patients may develop extensive scarring or chronic radiation dermatitis (itching, scaling, and change in pigmentation).

Follow-up for squamous cell cancer is particularly important because this type of cancer has a greater tendency than basal cell cancer to spread locally and to distant sites.

Testicle

Testicular cancers are rare. However, they are among the most common cancers affecting young men. Testicular tumors, which are non-tender, firm masses, are usually discovered first by the patient. Two major types of testicular cancer are recognized. The first is known as seminoma; the second is categorized as non-seminomatous cancer. Only seminomas will be discussed here, because they are often curable with radiation therapy. Non-seminomatous cancers are usually treated with chemotherapy.

TREATMENT. Following a biopsy that confirms the presence of cancer, surgery is performed. The testicle, its attachments, and the local lymph nodes are removed. (Human beings have thousands of lymph nodes, which act as filters for elements foreign to the body—infection and cancer, for example. Because they are so widely distributed throughout the body, lymph nodes often are affected when cancer begins to spread from its original site to adjacent tissues.)

There is generally a step-by-step progression of seminomas from the testicle to adjacent lymph nodes. These lymph nodes extend from the pelvis to the abdomen and then into the chest. Radiation therapy is administered to treat the lymph-node pathways of the pelvis and abdomen, and is performed following surgery. Should cancer be discovered to have spread to the lymph nodes of the abdomen, then radiation may also be given to those in the chest.

Seminomatous cancers are very sensitive to radiation, and only 2,000 to 3,000 units of radiation may be required to cure the disease. This is usually given in two to three weeks. Treatments are usually administered through the front and the back of the body, and the remaining testicle is carefully shielded to protect it from the radiation.

Many lymph nodes are involved in treatment, particularly those situated adjacent to the major blood vessels of the pelvis and abdomen. Therefore, the treatment field is necessarily quite large.

SIDE EFFECTS. Radiation dosages may adversely affect the opposite normal testicle, in spite of appropriate shielding. Sperm counts and motility will generally be depressed, and radiation may also cause damage to genetic material (chromosomes). This can lead to infertility and may harm future offspring. Because of this, men are advised to store sperm before initiating treatments.

Because the total radiation doses are low, patients usually do not experience significant side effects. If mild nausea occurs, it can be controlled easily with medication. (I prefer Compazine.)

On rare occasions, bone marrow may be affected by radiation treatments, and the patient may show lowering of the blood count. Although this is the exception, weekly blood counts are obtained as a precaution.

FOLLOW-UP AND OUTLOOK. It is important that patients undergo regular follow-up tests. Chest x-rays and CT scans of the abdomen and pelvis are extremely important to determine whether residual disease exists or new disease has occurred. There are also specialized blood tests (known as tumor markers) that can indicate the presence of the cancer, evaluate the results of the treatment, and detect its recurrence.

Because of the extreme sensitivity of the tumor cells to radiation, the cure rate for this type of cancer is very high. And, if radiation therapy should fail to effect a complete cure, chemotherapy can be used to treat the residual disease. More advanced disease, such as that which has spread to the chest, is currently treated with chemotherapy, with additional radiation if some tumor remains.

Uterus

The uterus is the medical term for the womb; the outlet of the uterus that leads to the vagina is called the cervix. The cancers that originate in the uterus and cervix have different biological characteristics, and therefore, they require different treatments and are discussed separately.

The most common uterine cancer begins in the lining (endometrium) of the organ. Eventually it extends to the underlying muscle wall of the uterus, and it may extend to the cervix. If the cancer progresses to more advanced stages it will spread to the ovaries, the vagina, the bladder, the rectum, or other adjacent sites.

About 75 percent of patients have localized disease at the time of discovery. When the cancer is confined to the uterine wall, as is often the case, there is a relatively good chance for a cure.

TREATMENT. Treatment for endometrial cancer is highly individualized. However, surgery, in which the uterus, the fallopian tubes, and the ovaries are removed, is the mainstay of early and moderately advanced uterine cancer.

External radiation therapy is often used in patients who are at high risk for recurrent cancer after surgery. Specifically, these patients have aggressive cancer cell types, and the cancer has involved a good part of the uterine muscle wall, or has spread to the cervix, or is suspected or discovered to have spread to adjacent lymph nodes. (The human body has thousands of lymph nodes, which filter elements foreign to the body. Because they are so widely distributed, lymph nodes are often affected when cancer spreads from its original site.) The combination of radiation therapy and surgery provides the best survival rates. Radiation therapy is sometimes given before surgery; in other cases, it is done after surgery.

Whether done before or after surgery, external treatment may deliver 3,000 to 5,000 units of radiation on a daily basis over a period of four to five weeks. Treatments are usually given through a four-portal technique, that is, treating the front, the back, and the sides of the pelvis.

If it is clinically indicated, a radioactive source is inserted into the vagina where it stays for a few days. This is known as internal radiation therapy. This increases the local radiation dose to the upper third of the vagina, which is often a site of recurrent cancer. A hospital admission is necessary, because the radioactive material is inserted while the patient is under mild anesthesia.

During the period in which the radioactive source is in place, the woman is confined to bed. The radioactive material is very powerful and lethal to cancer cells, but not to the rest of the body. Some of the radioactive energy escapes beyond the body, and prolonged exposure could be hazardous to others. Therefore, every hospital has a policy of precautions needed to insure the safety of visitors and hospital staff. In essence, this results in iso-lation of the patient except for necessary visits by health-care providers.

Quite recently, an alternate method of administering inter-nal radiation has been introduced in the United States, although it has already gained wide popularity in Europe and Asia. The method involves inserting the radioactive sources in rapid, high doses. The treatment is delivered on an outpatient basis, thus avoiding the complications and cost associated with general anesthetic and a hospital stay. Satisfactory results have been achieved with five treatments, which are combined with exter-nal radiation therapy. It has been demonstrated that this rapid, high-dose method is as effective as the traditional low-dose treatment previously described.

Some patients are not able to undergo surgery because their health does not allow it or because of the stage of their disease, and radiation therapy will be their only treatment. Radiation therapy has been found to be effective in both curing and con-trolling this cancer, but not as effective as when combined with surgery. Patients who receive only radiation are usually given external treatment first, followed by internal treatment to both the uterus and the vagina.

Patients are considered to have very advanced cancer when it has spread out of the uterus to the adjacent organs and pelvic tissues. These patients are treated with radiation therapy only, or they are given hormonal therapy or chemotherapy in addition to radiation. The goal is to palliate—that is, to arrest the disease and make the patient more comfortable.

SIDE EFFECTS. The side effects of *internal* treatment are moder-ate rectal and bladder irritation, which are controlled with med-ication. Generally speaking, patients are not in too much pain during this treatment because mild narcotic medication is prescribed. Internal radiation treatment may be performed in two sessions, requiring two hospital admissions.

Most women treated with *external* radiation are able to tolerate the treatments quite well, and side effects, while annoying, are not of serious concern. Most women who develop this type of cancer are beyond childbearing years, and the emotional response to losing the uterus may not be as significant as in younger women. (Seventy-five percent of uterine cancer occurs after age 50.)

External radiation treatments result in only mild to moderate side effects, including some diarrhea, urinary frequency, and mild reddening of the skin over the areas being treated. These symptoms usually begin within the second or third week of treatment. All symptoms can be easily controlled with appropriate medication. Diarrhea can be treated with Lomotil or Imodium A-D; urinary frequency is treated with medications such as Pyridium and Ditropan; skin irritation is treated with soothing skin creams (I generally recommend Nivea) and cortisone ointments.

FOLLOW-UP AND OUTLOOK. After treatment is completed, a woman is evaluated periodically by a gynecologist because it is absolutely essential that the pelvis and the vagina be checked for recurrent cancer. Chest x-rays, CT scans of the pelvis, and IVP examinations may be ordered to check for recurrent disease (see chapter 9).

Chapter 6

Radiation Therapy When Cancer Has Spread

I N THE PREVIOUS chapter I discussed treatment of *primary* cancers—that is, those originating in specific organs. This section deals with the treatment of cancers once they have traveled from the organ of origin to a distant site. This spread of disease is technically known as *metastasis* (the term also refers to the secondary growth itself). There is an in-between stage in which cancers invade the tissues surrounding the site of origin. This is referred to as *local invasion*.

Cancers begin as a cluster of cells multiplying in an out-of-control manner, unlike the body's normal cycle of cell destruction and replenishment. Particular abnormal genes (oncogenes) that influence this uncontrolled growth have been identified in some cancer cells.

Scientists believe that once a cluster of cancer cells has arisen in an organ, there is a step-by-step progressive pattern in cancer growth and spread. At first, the body's immune system resists the growth of the invader, a process that may take years. Once the battle tips in favor of the cancer, local growth proceeds. At some point, and this point is thought to vary among cancers as well as individuals, the cancer spreads locally into the surrounding tissues. The next step is for cancer cells to attach themselves to and penetrate the neighboring blood-vessel and lymph-vessel walls.

Once the cancer cells have penetrated the blood-vessel wall, they enter the bloodstream and the lymph system of the body. Cells traveling in the lymph system settle in the lymph nodes. The cancer cells then travel throughout the body, but must reattach to and penetrate the vessel wall at a distant site. The organs into which these cells settle are generally those richly endowed with blood vessels and with nutrient materials. Thus, the bones, the liver, the lungs, and the brain are common sites for metastases.

Future improvement in cancer therapy will occur when scientists discover chemicals that prevent metastases by blocking the attachment and penetration of cancer cells to blood and lymph vessels. It is these metastases that often represent the failure to cure cancers, because most distant metastases are invariably fatal. Thus, many patients whose primary cancers are cured die because of the effects of distant metastases to the brain, lungs, and/or liver, where cure rates are negligible. However, metastases to bones in and of themselves may not be fatal and are often cured. Unfortunately, many cancers affect not only the bone but vital organs as well, and deaths occur from the effects to these organs in spite of the cure of bone metastases.

When radiation therapy (or chemotherapy or surgery) is administered to metastases, we generally refer to it as *palliative* treatment. This means that we are attempting to control the disease by relieving symptoms such as pain, neurological problems, and the effects of pressure on vital organs, rather than curing the disease.

Many patients undergoing radiation therapy for metastases have previously undergone radiation treatment and other cancer therapy for their primary disease. The treatments to the primary disease are usually administered before we know that metastases have occurred. Simply put, the primary disease may have been cured while the coexisting metastases went undetected. In spite of today's sophisticated technology, many metastases are not diagnosed because of their small size. Therefore, a significant number of patients may be cured of their local disease only to be seen for further treatment for metastases at distant sites months or years later.

Another group of patients receiving radiation therapy for metastases are those with a coexisting primary cancer, meaning that both cancers have been discovered at the same time. Treatment may then be delivered to both areas simultaneously or in sequence. Depending on the clinical situation, only one area may be treated. In other words, metastases may be treated without also treating the primary cancer. We do this because metastases may cause more clinal problems than the primary tumor. For example, lung cancer that has spread to the brain may create many neurological difficulties, while the primary tumor in the lung is silent, that is, it produces no symptoms. Similarly, metastatic tumors in the bone cause pain and loss of motion, while the primary cancer is not causing discomfort. A judgment must then be made about how aggressively to treat the primary disease. Alleviating the patient's suffering takes precedence over treating the primary cancer.

Physicians sometimes use combination treatment, such as chemotherapy to treat the primary disease and radiation to treat the metastases. Radiation is usually delivered when cancers have spread to the bone, brain, chest, lymph nodes, skin, and spine, each of which is discussed below.

Bone

Over 50 percent of patients with breast, lung, and prostate cancer develop metastases to the bone. Other primary cancers may also spread to the bone, but this occurs less frequently.

The symptoms that patients experience include pain and limited motion caused by destruction of the bone and/or stretching of associated nerve fibers. (Although the vertebrae of the spine are considered bone, I have included a separate section on the spine because the spinal cord and its nerves warrant individual discussion.)

TREATMENT. The amount of radiation delivered to skeletal areas depends on the size of the disease and its location. Radiation therapy is usually the most effective and rapid way to relieve bone pain caused by cancer. (Hormonal therapy for breast and prostate cancer metastases to the bone can be very effective, and it is generally recommended when the cancer in the bones is widespread.) The pain is completely alleviated in 75 to 90 percent of cases, depending on the site of the original disease. The amount of radiation and duration of treatment is guided by the alleviation of pain. However, clinical experience allows the radiation therapist to predict fairly accurately how quickly and completely a metastatic cancer will respond to a particular schedule of treatment. Therefore, depending on where the cancer originated, bones affected by cancer will require differing amounts of radiation over variable periods of time.

Weight-bearing bones of the leg often require more radiation than non-weight-bearing bones. When more than one-third of the width of one of these long bones is affected, it is weakened to the point where fractures could occur. When your physicians suspect that such a fracture will take place, an orthopedic device (a metal rod) may be inserted. This procedure limits further damage to the bone and provides pain relief. Radiation therapy is started after the orthopedic procedure is performed.

The patient has an important role in helping the radiation therapist design an area of treatment. The area of bone pain generally corresponds quite accurately to the site of the disease. Physical examination will also help determine the areas to be treated. X-rays and nuclear bone scans (see chapter 9) are extremely helpful in designing the portal to be used. The diminishing pain is usually a reliable indicator that cancer in the area being treated has been destroyed.

In general, excellent results will be achieved after 10 to 15 treatments delivered over a period of two to three weeks. This relatively short treatment time, in which the radiation therapist delivers a high dose of radiation, is possible because bones of the arms and legs can tolerate a higher dose of radiation than, for example, the more sensitive soft tissues of the abdomen. Because of the adjacent soft tissues, the bones of the spine, skull, and pelvis are treated less rapidly.

The patient's response will help guide the exact level of the dosage, and the radiation therapist notes subsiding pain and return of motion to the affected structures. Once a sufficient dose of radiation has been delivered to a particular area, it is unlikely that the pain and disease will return to the same location.

A total dose of 3,000 to 5,000 units of radiation is usually sufficient; the average is about 4,000 units.

Bone pain disappears because the cancer in the bone has been eradicated or its growth arrested by the radiation treatments. As a rule, pain decreases within the first two weeks of treatment, and it may begin to subside after the first few treatments. The response varies among individuals, but the greatest variation depends upon the primary site of the cancer. For example, bones affected by prostate cancers generally respond quickly to radiation therapy within the first two weeks. Bones affected by lung cancer may take longer to improve, and the response of bones affected by breast cancer is somewhere in between. However, response also varies among individuals with the same cancer. Therefore, there is no hard-and-fast rule concerning how quickly pain will be relieved.

Patients tend to fall into one of four pain-response groups. The first are patients who have immediate pain relief, often beginning within a week or two after treatment is initiated. The second group includes patients who obtain relief toward the end of the treatment course. In the third group are patients, fortunately in the minority, who do not get pain relief until several weeks after treatment is completed. Approximately 5 to 10 percent of patients never experience sufficient pain relief. In my experience, these patients require continued pain medication or a surgical procedure to block the nerve fibers responsible for the pain.

As pain lessens, patients describe it as changing from sharp to dull. Mobility of the affected area improves, and patients experience psychological relief as well. They look and feel better and are able to follow a more normal lifestyle because of their renewed feeling of well-being. Sleep patterns usually return to normal; appetite improves. Many people are able to eliminate pain medication, and even those taking strong narcotics are able to reduce the dosage or switch to over-the-counter pain-relief medications.

Care is taken not to treat too many bones simultaneously, because radiation may affect the bone marrow's ability to manufacture blood cells.

SIDE EFFECTS. The side effects encountered when delivering radiation to the bones vary greatly, depending on the location of the bones being treated. There are generally no side effects from radiation treatments to the long bones of the arms and legs because the soft tissues in the path of the radiation beam do not react.

Side effects are experienced when the bones being treated are those lying next to sensitive organs. For example, treating pelvic bones will result in radiation to the intestines, which may cause diarrhea and nausea. Treating the bones of the neck will affect the esophagus (swallowing tube), causing sore throat and difficulty in swallowing. These side effects are temporary and can be controlled with medication and dietary modifications. They usually disappear within a week or two after radiation treatment has been completed.

FOLLOW-UP AND OUTLOOK. Follow-up x-rays and nuclear bone scans (see chapter 9) often reveal improvement because the cancer has been destroyed or arrested. These tests are also used to detect new areas of disease.

Brain

The radiation treatment described here is that given to patients whose original cancer has spread (metastasized) to the brain. (See chapter 5 for an explanation of the radiation treatment that is delivered when the brain is the site of the *primary* cancer.) Your radiation therapist will design the treatment field after reviewing tests (generally CT and MRI scans) that reveal the location of the metastatic disease (see chapter 9). However, in most cases, the entire brain is treated, because metastatic disease usually produces multiple tumors. Even when only one or two tumor deposits are revealed in the imaging tests, physicians generally believe that additional disease is present but the deposits are too small to be imaged. Therefore, treatment portals are designed to include all the important areas that need radiation treatment.

Currently, clinical trials show that surgery for some types of brain metastases can prolong survival, although it does not cure the disease. (Chemotherapy is generally not recommended for metastatic disease occurring in the brain, because it has not been shown to improve quality of life or affect survival.)

TREATMENT. A patient's clinical situation will affect the total dose of radiation administered as well as the length of treatment. Some cancer specialists favor rapid high-dose treatment (approximately 3,000 units in two and a half weeks), and others favor treatment doses administered over a longer period of time (approximately 5,000 units in five and a half weeks). However, the extent of the disease in the brain, the site of the primary cancer, and the patient's overall condition are the major considerations when the treatment plan is designed.

Cortisone medication is given along with radiation therapy to reduce the swelling of the brain tissues, a condition called edema. The edema is often caused by the tumors, but it may also be aggravated by the radiation treatments. Anticonvulsant medications are also often prescribed.

Clinical trials are currently under way to test the use of a technique called radio surgery in treating metastatic tumors of the brain. Radio surgery is performed infrequently because it is practical when only one tumor appears in the brain. The tumor is exposed during a surgical procedure, and high-energy radiation is delivered to the affected area. This is still an experimental technique, however, and appropriate in a very limited number of cases.

SIDE EFFECTS. Two common side effects of radiation to the brain are drowsiness and disorientation, sometimes occurring one to two hours after treatment. For this reason, I usually advise patients to sleep and rest after each treatment. These symptoms can be alarming to the patient because, quite naturally, people associate the brain with the functions that make them alert and able to participate in life. However, there is no medical cause for concern, and mental functioning returns to normal after a short period of time. Some patients experience mild nausea and headaches, both of which can be controlled with medication. Fatigue may begin some time during treatment. Nausea can be alleviated with Compazine, headaches with over-the-counter pain-relief medications.

Severe headaches, projectile vomiting, and vision changes are rare symptoms, but when they occur they signal an increase in pressure inside the brain. Radiation therapy may be temporarily stopped or the dosage of cortisone medication increased.

Hair loss can cause a significant emotional side effect. The amount of hair loss is related to the amount of radiation given; the higher the dose, the more likely the hair loss. Generally, an excess of 3,000 units (a very common dose) will result in some hair loss, but only in the area receiving the treatment. Although some people do not experience hair loss because of especially strong hair follicles, patients should expect it and prepare for it in advance. I advise my patients to obtain a hairpiece before any loss occurs. In this way, they will never undergo a period of baldness, and a sense of self and body image can be preserved.

Hair loss usually starts about two weeks after the beginning of treatment, and in many cases the hair will not grow back. For those whose hair does grow back, the new growth is usually sparse and the texture is altered. If smaller areas are treated, rather than the whole brain, then hair loss will occur only at the site receiving radiation. The scalp may become irritated, and a skin cream (I prefer Nivea) will usually alleviate the discomfort.

FOLLOW-UP AND OUTLOOK. When radiation is administered to the brain for metastatic disease, it is considered palliative, in that it temporarily arrests the growth of the cancer and relieves pain. Unfortunately, cures are rare.

Six to eight weeks following completion of radiation therapy, MRI and CT scans are performed to evaluate results (see chapter 9).

Chest

Metastases to the chest, which includes the lung and its covering (known as the pleura), and rib cage can cause a variety of symptoms. These include pain, pressure, bleeding, and shortness of breath. When metastases involve the rib cage, pain is the usual symptom. Radiation therapy is very effective in rapidly reducing bone pain. Chest x-rays and CT scans (see chapter 9) are performed to locate the areas of disease and to follow up on the results of treatment.

TREATMENT. A dose of 3,000 to 4,000 units may be delivered over two to three weeks and is usually sufficient to alleviate rib pain.

When metastatic cancers occur in the area between the lungs (mediastinum), obstruction of the breathing passages (bronchial tubes) may occur. A short course of radiation therapy to the affected area generally relieves the shortness of breath and any bleeding or pain. A total dose of 3,000 to 4,000 units of radiation may be delivered over a period of about three to four weeks.

In some situations, radiation therapy is of limited value in treating metastatic cancer in the chest area. Fluid around the lung (pleural effusion) and fluid around the heart (pericardial effusion) do not respond well to radiation. Chemotherapy and surgical procedures (removal of the fluid with a needle) will be temporarily effective. Radiation therapy has not been shown to be of much value for treating multiple metastases in the lungs. Depending on the type of primary cancer, chemotherapy may be effective for this condition.

SIDE EFFECTS. When small areas of the ribs or pleura are being treated, there are generally no side effects. However, when larger areas of the chest are treated, the patient may experience some nausea, which can be controlled with Compazine.

FOLLOW-UP AND OUTLOOK. Radiation is usually very effective in alleviating pain and bleeding; results are not as good for relieving obstruction. There is also great variation in patients' response to treatment. Chest x-rays and CT scans are very accurate in evaluating the results of radiation therapy.

Lymph Nodes

Cancer discovered in lymph nodes has metastasized from a primary site. Although Hodgkin's disease and non-Hodgkin's lymphomas are thought to originate in the lymph nodes, the presence of these cancers in many lymph nodes can be considered metastases, because the disease has spread from one lymph node to another.

The human body contains thousands of lymph nodes, distributed throughout the body. The lymph nodes are part of the lymphatic system, which is a component of the body's immune system. Lymph nodes filter foreign elements in the body—infections and cancer, for example.

Physicians can evaluate, by touch and sight, lymph nodes that are close to the surface of the body. Those that are suspicious for cancer can then be biopsied to confirm the diagnosis. Lymph nodes that lie deep in the body require imaging tests, such as CT and MRI scans, to detect and evaluate possible cancers. Lymph nodes that contain cancer do not usually cause pain unless an infection exists concurrently. As a rule, large lymph nodes that contain cancer are more difficult to cure than small lymph nodes.

TREATMENT. The path of lymph-node involvement in various cancers is often predictable, and treatment plans are designed according to what is known about each pathway of spread. (There are *notable exceptions* to this, which cancer specialists take into consideration when they design treatment plans.) Radiation therapy dosages for lymph nodes vary according to the origin of the cancer and the size of the lymph node being treated. Therefore, cancerous lymph nodes from prostate cancer will require a different dose than cancerous lymph nodes caused by Hodgkin's lymphoma.

Radiation treatments to lymph nodes often begin at the time the primary cancer is discovered if it is *suspected*, though not yet proven, that the lymph nodes are cancerous. It is also delivered to lymph nodes when imaging tests such as CT or MRI scans identify lymph-node enlargement considered to be caused by cancer. Radiation therapy is also commonly performed after surgery has removed the primary cancer and it is *proven* that the lymph nodes contain cancer.

Lymph nodes may require additional re-treatment if the original radiation therapy was unsuccessful. Chemotherapy may later be added. For some cancers, particularly the lymphomas, chemotherapy is often the *initial* treatment and radiation follows to treat residual disease.

For clarity, I will discuss lymph-node treatment in groups, starting at the top of the body.

As a rule, cancers originating in the *brain* do not spread to lymph nodes, and therefore radiation treatment is delivered only to the primary site. Cancers of the head and neck can spread to the local lymph nodes of the neck. Surgery is often performed to remove these metastases, and is followed by radiation or chemotherapy. Disease in these lymph nodes can often be evaluated by sight and touch; lymph nodes located deeper in the tissues are evaluated by CT or MRI scans.

Lymph nodes of the *head and neck* are often difficult to cure because of their size and number at the time the cancer is discovered. Moreover, it is often the appearance of these lymph nodes that first suggests that an undiscovered cancer is present in the area. The size and number of lymph nodes, as well as the cancer's natural resistance to being easily destroyed, means that radiation treatment portals will be large and the dosages high. In addition, infections often exist in these lymph-node metastases and must be treated with antibiotics.

Breast cancer will often metastasize to local lymph nodes. The underarm region, known as the axilla, is the most frequent, and often the first, site of spread. Generally, it is necessary to biopsy the lymph nodes to determine if cancer is present, although if they are large, the lymph nodes may be detected through a physical examination. Breast cancer may also spread to lymph nodes in the chest wall, behind the breast, and beneath the breast bone. As a rule, lymph nodes in these areas can be neither imaged nor felt. Therefore, radiation and chemotherapy are administered when the presence of cancer is likely. Enough information is known about the spread of the disease to establish a degree of probability that can help guide treatment decisions. The tendency for the cancer to spread to adjacent lymph-node groups is one reason that radiation therapy for breast cancer requires a large treatment field.

Cancer of the *lung and esophagus* will usually spread to lymph nodes in the chest, and it may also extend to the lower neck and upper abdomen. The deep lymph nodes of the chest can be evaluated only by imaging tests such as x-rays and MRI and CT scans (see chapter 9). In my experience, the CT scan is the most effective test for this purpose because the number and size of lymph nodes are shown in great detail. Treatment can then be planned to include all the chains of diseased lymph nodes that are discovered on the CT scan.

By the time they are discovered, many lung and esophageal cancers have already spread to the nearby lymph-node groups, which is why radiation treatment portals are large. Both the primary cancer and the adjacent lymph nodes can be treated simultaneously.

Cancers of the *pancreas* rapidly spread to the adjacent lymph-node groups, which then require radiation treatment. These lymph nodes are deep within the body, and a CT scan is the best way to evaluate them for disease.

Treatment of cancers in the *pelvic region*—the prostate, uterus, cervix, bladder, testicle, and rectosigmoid colon— usually includes the lymph nodes next to the organ that contains the primary cancer. At the time these cancers are discovered, they may have already spread to the surrounding lymph-node groups. The treatment portals will be large, allowing the primary cancer and the nearby lymph nodes to be treated simultaneously. Chemotherapy is of additional value in treating lymph-node cancers in this region, particularly testicular and colon cancers.

Cancers that are thought to originate in lymph nodes (Hodgkin's disease and non-Hodgkin's lymphoma) spread from one group, or "chain," of lymph nodes to another. The radiation doses needed to cure or control these lymph-node cancers are not usually as high as those delivered for other cancers. However, the area being treated is large in order to include all the lymph nodes that are potentially affected by the cancer. This is particularly true in the case of Hodgkin's disease, where, for example, a known lymph-node cancer in one side of the neck will require that lymph-node groups in both sides of the neck, the underarm area, and the chest be included in the treatment (see chapter 5).

SIDE EFFECTS. The side effects of radiation therapy directed to lymph nodes correspond to the area of the body being treated. For example, when radiation is directed to the pelvic region, side effects may include cramping, diarrhea, and urinary frequency and urgency. Treatment to the upper abdomen primarily causes nausea and indigestion. Refer to chapter 2 for a discussion of expected side effects and their treatment.

FOLLOW-UP AND OUTLOOK. Results of treatment are evaluated by physical examination if the lymph nodes are close to the surface of the body. The lymph nodes should shrink to a very small size after radiation therapy. However, they generally do not completely disappear because scar tissue forms and is felt as a small nodule. If physicians suspect that cancer still remains in a lymph node, it is necessary to physically monitor changes in the lymph node over a prolonged period of time, or a biopsy may be required.

Lymph nodes that are located deep in the body can be evaluated only by imaging tests. Size and number should decrease following either radiation or chemotherapy, and periodic testing will show whether the treatments were effective. On occasion, it may be necessary to perform a biopsy to confirm that the disease has been arrested. In certain cases, lymphangiograms (see chapter 9) may be helpful in evaluating the results of treatment.

Metastases to the lymph nodes is generally the second step of cancer progression after the initial growth. Although there are exceptions, the next step is generally dissemination throughout the body. Therefore, lymph-node metastases should be treated aggressively, especially when a cure is considered possible.

Skin

Metastases to the chest wall (skin and underlying soft tissues) may occur months or years following a mastectomy for breast cancer. Radiation is used to treat this metastatic disease, which is not necessarily life threatening. However, skin metastases resulting from other kinds of cancer, such as lung cancer, are generally considered to be a sign of very advanced disease. Ten to 20 percent of patients who have had a radical or modified radical mastectomy experience metastases to the skin. This is referred to as *local* disease because the chest wall and breast are in the same location. When the breast cancer is more advanced at the time of diagnosis, the percentages of skin metastases are higher. While the situation is serious, it is by no means hopeless.

TREATMENT. Many patients who develop these local recurrences but show no evidence of distant metastases have a relatively good overall prognosis. If these cancerous lesions are left untreated, they will progress into painful, infected ulcerations. One or two local deposits may be easily surgically removed. However, when multiple deposits are present, as is often the case, radiation therapy is delivered to the entire chest wall to prevent later problems with ulceration, bleeding, and pain. Approximately 5,000 units of radiation are delivered to the entire chest wall in five to six weeks. Most patients are seen during the early stage and cured of their local disease. Patients with more advanced disease may require different dose and time schedules. Radiation may still help heal the ulcers, stop the bleeding, and arrest the infection. Many radiation therapists advocate treating the entire chest wall as soon as even one metastatic growth develops, because of the probability that cancers will appear in other areas.

SIDE EFFECTS. These radiation treatments do not cause significant side effects, except for mild reddening of the skin, more common among fair-skinned individuals. Occasionally, patients develop scarring of that portion of the lung which, despite efforts to keep exposure to a minimum, has received some radiation.

Some patients may develop an inflammation of the lung tissue (pneumonitis), which is treated with cortisone and sometimes antibiotics.

OUTLOOK. Depending on the stage of the cancer, radiation therapy administered to the chest wall immediately after the mastectomy or lumpectomy will reduce the incidence of skin recurrences. Women developing skin metastases shortly after surgery (within a year or two) do not have as good five-year survival rates as those whose skin metastases occur two years or longer after surgery.

Spine

The spine consists of seven vertebrae in the neck (the cervical area), twelve in the upper and middle back (the thoracic area), five in the lower back (the lumbar region), and approximately ten in the tailbone (sacrum and coccyx). The bony vertebrae enclose the spinal cord and the nerves that exit from it. The spinal cord, originating in the upper neck, is connected to the lower part of the brain and ends at the lower thoracic vertebrae. The spinal cord is bathed by spinal fluid and is surrounded and contained by a membrane known as the dura.

Tumors may spread to the vertebral bone or to the spaces around the dura, or to both areas simultaneously. When the bone is involved, pain and limited motion are frequent symptoms. When the dural spaces are involved, with or without bone involvement, a common result is loss of motor or sensory function. These symptoms occur because as the tumor enlarges, it creates pressure on the spinal cord and the adjacent nerves. How much motor or sensory function is lost depends on the tumor's location and the extent to which the spinal cord and nerves are involved. Most cancers can extend to the spine; however, lung, breast, prostate cancers, and lymphomas are the most likely primary cancers to affect this region of the body.

A variety of tests may be used to evaluate the extent of the disease. For example, bone x-rays may reveal bone destruction, which often results in fractures of the vertebrae. A nuclear bone scan is a very sensitive means of detecting bone metastases. CT and MRI scans (see chapter 9) may also be performed to further evaluate the extent of the disease, particularly when the cancer involves the dural tissues around the spinal cord.

TREATMENT. When it is found that *only* bone tissue is involved in the disease, radiation therapy is given to reduce pain, improve limited motion, and prevent further spread of the cancer to the spinal cord and adjacent nerves. A dose of 3,000 to 5,000 units of radiation may be delivered over a two- to four-week period. The total dosage and treatment time depend on how quickly the pain disappears, the origin of the primary cancer, the extent of the disease, and the patient's overall physical condition. Most patients experience significant pain relief.

Cancer involving the spinal cord and nerves (with or without bone disease) may result in one of the few radiation-therapy emergencies. The loss of nerve function must be treated immediately; if it is not, normal function will not return. A short course of radiation with relatively high daily doses is often necessary to reduce acute symptoms. The exact level of radiation and the total daily dose are tailored to the cancer's site of origin, the extent of the disease, and the patient's response to treatment. In addition to radiation therapy, cortisone medication (prednisone or Decadron) is given simultaneously to help relieve pressure on the spinal cord caused by swelling of the tissues.

On occasion, some bone tissue is surgically removed to relieve pressure on the spinal cord (laminectomy). Radiation therapy is then administered to treat the remaining tumor deposits.

SIDE EFFECTS. The location of the disease will determine the kind of side effects experienced. Radiation therapy to the cervical vertebrae may cause throat pain; radiation delivered to the mid-back may cause nausea and heartburn; radiation to the lower spine may cause nausea and diarrhea. These side effects occur because as the radiation beam goes through the spine, the soft tissues of the neck, chest, and abdomen are in its path. (For further discussion of side effects, see chapter 2.)

OUTLOOK. If neurological symptoms are caught *early* (within approximately 12 hours), radiation treatment may reverse the damage in many patients or halt its progress. This is the reason that delivering radiation therapy to the spine is often considered urgent. Unfortunately, the treatment is not always effective, no matter how aggressive the effort, and the patient's symptoms will progress. In other cases, the cancer is detected too late for treatments to be effective. These patients will experience varying degrees of neurologic impairment that is not reversible.

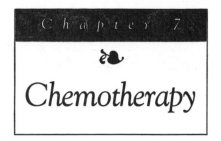

Chapter 7

Chemotherapy

CHEMOTHERAPY, THE treatment of cancer with anticancer drugs, can be administered before or after radiation therapy; in certain situations, it is given in conjunction with radiation treatments. The timing and duration of either treatment involves a complex series of decisions made after test results, the individual's age and physical condition, and other relevant factors have been considered. *Therefore, the information about chemotherapy presented here is by necessity basic and general.* Your *chemotherapist* can answer questions about the specific action of the drug you are given, as well as the temporary or long-term side effects you may experience.

Chemotherapy is distinguished from radiation and surgery, which are local treatments, in that it involves treatment of cancer by agents that circulate through the entire body by flowing through the bloodstream. Some chemicals are administered by mouth; others are injected directly into blood vessels. In a small number of cases, treatments are administered into other areas of the body—the abdominal and pelvic cavities, for example—rather than the blood vessels. Chemotherapy is often referred to as *systemic* treatment, meaning that the entire body is affected by the drug. Thus, the chemotherapeutic agent reaches *all* the cells of the body.

An unfortunate consequence of chemotherapy is that normal cells in the *whole* body are affected along with the cancerous cells. The effectiveness of chemotherapy is evaluated by the extent to which the chemicals are able to *selectively* alter the reproduction of tumor cells. The alteration of cancer cells needs to be powerful and long-lasting while having as few adverse effects as possible on the normal cells of the body.

Chemotherapy is prescribed for the treatment of cancer *originating* in an organ (the primary tumor); for the treatment of cancer that has spread to another organ or organs (metastatic disease); and for the treatment of disease that may be in the body but has not yet been detected, a treatment known as *adjuvant* chemotherapy.

AN EVOLVING TREATMENT

Chemotherapy is in constant change; old drugs are being discarded as scientists develop new drugs that are both more effective and less toxic to the body. Of the three major cancer treatments—chemotherapy, surgery, and radiation—it is chemotherapy that is currently in the greatest transition. This is why it's so difficult to make definitive statements about a particular drug for a specific cancer. What is true today may not be true tomorrow.

A few drugs remain a standard part of common treatment plans because their effectiveness has been well established. Major improvements have been made in chemotherapeutic treatments, resulting in higher cure rates, for childhood acute lymphocytic leukemia, Hodgkin's disease and some non-Hodgkin's lymphomas, testicular and ovarian cancers.

Chemotherapy may be given as a single agent (one chemical) or in combination. Combination treatments are often the most effective, because tumor cells generally do not behave uniformly in the same patient. When chemicals are combined it is possible to destroy different cells in the same cancer. Tumor cells may also mutate. This means that they change their biologic behavior, thereby altering their susceptibility to the chemotherapeutic agents. A combination of chemicals is more effective in destroying those cells that are altered. The resistance of cells to chemotherapy helps explain why this mode of treatment may *not* eradicate all cancer cells in a particular patient. Thus, treatment may fail and the cancer progresses.

Many factors are taken into consideration when oncologists plan chemotherapy treatments. Increased cancer-cell resistance, tumor-cell variation in the same patient, and the side effects and injury to the body caused by the chemicals themselves are evaluated. There must be a reasonable hope that this chemical assault on the body will be offset by an increased possibility of long-term survival.

SIDE EFFECTS OF CHEMOTHERAPY

Most chemotherapeutic agents have side effects that are at the very least annoying and at worst quite severe. These symptoms may be aggravated when radiation therapy is delivered in conjunction with chemotherapy. Your team of physicians can prescribe medications and give you advice about diet and lifestyle changes that will help alleviate these side effects. You should report symptoms as soon as they appear—there is no need to suffer in silence. While some side effects are best treated by your oncologist, if radiation is being administered in conjunction with chemotherapy you should also report symptoms to your radiation therapist. Although your radiation therapist will consult with the chemotherapist about these medications, it helps if you are familiar with the names of the chemicals that you are receiving.

The drugs listed below interact with radiation therapy, especially if the radiation is administered to the digestive tract. Nausea, vomiting, and loss of appetite are primary side effects of chemotherapy. However, it is unusual to discontinue chemotherapy or radiation as a result of intestinal side effects because they often can be effectively controlled with medication. When drugs that create irritation to the mouth, the esophagus, or the intestinal passage are used, radiation treatments are administered with special care because these symptoms are often aggravated.

Most of these drugs also reduce the ability of bone marrow to manufacture blood cells (white cells, red cells, and platelets). When a significant portion of bone marrow is irradiated, the effects on the blood count will be more severe. If a blood test known as the complete blood count (CBC) reveals that these cells are significantly reduced in number, both chemotherapy and radiation treatments may have to be modified or even discontinued for a period of time. New drugs are currently being developed to stimulate the bone marrow and reduce this side effect.

Decreases in red blood cells result in less oxygen being received by the tissues. Patients may then feel weaker and more fatigued. The decrease in oxygen may also significantly affect the heart and brain, a situation that can have serious consequences. Blood transfusions may be required to increase the red blood-cell count.

Decreases in white blood-cell count will lead to increased susceptibility to infection. Treatments may be interrupted to allow the white blood-cell numbers to return to normal. New drugs are being developed (some are already in use) that will stimulate the white blood-cell production.

Chemotherapy may also cause a decrease in platelets, resulting in bleeding due to altered clotting ability. This decrease in platelets can be corrected by transfusions or simply by allowing time for the count to return to normal.

In some cases, it becomes necessary to temporarily suspend chemotherapy, radiation treatment, or both. A break in treatment gives the bone marrow time to reconstitute itself and increase the white blood cells and platelets in the bloodstream. Again, new drugs that stimulate the bone marrow may lessen the need to temporarily stop treatment.

Other side effects of chemotherapy vary from agent to agent, and I urge you to refer to books specifically about chemotherapy (see the reading list on page 200).

SOME CHEMOTHERAPEUTIC DRUGS

In the following list, the brand name is bold, the generic name is in parentheses, because patients usually refer to the drug by its brand name. When discussing the use of these drugs, I have included only those cancers mentioned in this book. Many chemotherapeutic agents are used for a variety of cancers not mentioned. While the list of drugs is not complete, it includes the drugs often used in conjunction with radiation. Thus, you will be made aware of situations in which radiation and chemo-therapy interact.

In reviewing the following commonly administered drugs, I will outline typical side effects and explain how those symptoms may be affected by radiation therapy. A more comprehensive list of these drugs, including detailed descriptions of their uses and side effects, can be found in books on chemotherapy.

ADRIAMYCIN (Doxorubicin) is a common agent used to treat bladder, breast, and lung cancers as well as Hodgkin's disease and non-Hodgkin's lymphoma. The gastrointestinal side effects experienced are generally nausea, vomiting, mouth irritation, and diarrhea. The bone marrow may be affected and the blood count lowered. This drug also can affect the heart rhythm and may cause the heart to enlarge, reducing its ability to function properly. Heart failure may also occur because the drug results in enlargement of the heart. Hair loss is common, but regrowth may occur several months after treatment is completed.

Cardiac changes may be aggravated if radiation therapy is delivered to the chest in conjunction with Adriamycin. If radia-tion treatments are directed to the abdomen or over large areas of the body, gastrointestinal side effects and bone-marrow changes may be aggravated as well.

CARMUSTINE (BCNU) is used to treat brain tumors, multiple myeloma, Hodgkin's disease, and non-Hodgkin's lymphoma. Nausea and vomiting may begin several hours after the drug is administered, and liver function may be altered. BCNU also results in a decrease of white blood cells and platelets. Unlike other drugs, BCNU crosses into the brain tissue when adminis-tered. Therefore, it is often used for treatment of brain tumors following radiation therapy. This drug does not appear to aggra-vate the side effects of radiation.

BLENOXANE (Bleomycin) can be used for Hodgkin's disease, non-Hodgkin's lymphoma, testicular cancer, and cancers of the cervix and of the head and neck. Nausea, vomiting, and irrita-tion of the lining of the mouth are common side effects. Patients may also experience allergic reactions to the drug, resulting in fever, chills, a rise in temperature, and a drop in blood pressure. The skin on the hands and feet may peel, and there may be some change in skin color, ridging of the nails, and hair loss. This drug may affect the lungs and produce pneumonia or scarring of the lung tissues. Radiation therapy may aggravate these problems, and therefore, lung function must be monitored and chest x-rays taken.

CYTOXAN (Cyclophosphamide) can be used in the treatment of breast cancer, lung cancer, Hodgkin's disease, multiple myeloma, non-Hodgkin's lymphoma, and ovarian cancer. The side effects of cyclophosphamide include loss of appetite, nausea and vomiting, mouth irritation, anemia, and decrease of the white blood-cell count because of effects on the bone marrow. Nausea and vomiting usually begin about six hours after the drug is administered. The drug also affects the bladder, and some blood may appear in the urine. Hair loss, ridging of the nails, and pigment changes in the skin are also common side effects. Sperm production may drop in men, and women may experience changes in their menstrual cycles, including cessation of the monthly period. Although there is variation among patients' ability to tolerate the drug, these side effects are generally moderate to severe in intensity.

When radiation treatments and chemotherapy are administered during the same period or in close sequence, the digestive-system side effects may be exacerbated. In addition, the effects on the blood count may also be accentuated because both treatments affect the bone marrow.

5-FU (Fluorouracil) is commonly used for colon, rectal, gastric, and pancreatic cancers. Gastrointestinal side effects include loss of appetite, nausea and vomiting, and diarrhea. The lining of the mouth may also become irritated. The effect on bone marrow causes a decrease in white and red blood cells and platelets. Patients may also experience hair loss and skin irritation.

In the treatment of cancers of the digestive tract, radiation treatment is often delivered in conjunction with, or shortly

before or after 5-FU is administered. Because radiation treatments are delivered to the abdominal area, gastrointestinal side
effects may be accentuated.

METHOTREXATE (Amethopterin) is often used in treating cancers of the breast, lung, head, and neck, testicular cancers, and
non-Hodgkin's lymphoma. Common side effects include irritation of the lining of the mouth and diarrhea. Because some
damage to the liver and kidneys may occur, both liver and kidney
function are tested prior to treatment to evaluate any preexisting
conditions that could limit the use of chemotherapy. The drug
may affect the nervous system, and patients may experience
headaches, drowsiness, and blurred vision. Decreases in red and
white blood cells and platelets often occur because of the effects
on bone marrow. Radiation therapy can further lower the blood
count if the treatment fields are large and include extensive areas
of bone.

MUTAMYCIN (Mitomycin-C) can be used for breast, gastric,
lung, pancreatic, and colon and rectal cancers. Nausea, vomiting, loss of appetite, and hair loss are the usual side effects, along
with decreases in white and red blood-cell counts and platelets.
Radiation therapy can aggravate the effects on the blood count
and the intestinal side effects.

NITROGEN MUSTARD (Mechlorethamine) is often used for
treating Hodgkin's disease, non-Hodgkin's lymphoma, and cancerous fluid collections around the lungs (malignant pleural effusions). Nausea, vomitting, and loss of appetite often occur, as
well as a lowering of the blood count. Sterility may also result.
Radiation administered to treat the lymphomas may aggravate
these side effects.

ONCOVIN (Vincristine) can be used for breast cancer, Hodgkin's
disease, and non-Hodgkin's lymphoma and testicicular cancer.
Many side effects are neurologic in nature. They include abnormal feelings along the nerve pathways, numbness and tingling,
loss of balance, and changes in motor coordination. Constipation

and abdominal pain may also occur. Radiation to the abdomen may aggravate the pain.

PLATINOL (Cisplatin) can be used to treat bladder, lung, ovarian, cervical, and testicular cancers, as well as some cancers of the uterus, head, and neck. Severe nausea and vomiting usually occur. Loss of appetite and more mild nausea may persist for about a week after treatment. The kidneys may also be affected, and kidney function must be closely monitored. Other side effects include possible hearing loss (a new derivative drug, Paraplatin, has lessened this side effect), loss of motor function, and unusual sensations along the nerve pathways. Decreases in red and white blood cells and platelets also result from treatment with cisplatin.

Intravenous medication is often used to minimize the nausea and vomiting. When radiation is administered over areas of the digestive tract, it will aggravate all the drug's gastrointestinal side effects.

PROCARBAZINE (both generic and brand name) is commonly used to treat Hodgkin's disease. Nausea and vomiting often occur, as well as a lowering of the blood count. These side effects may be aggravated by radiation therapy.

VELBAN (Vinblastine) can be commonly used for breast and testicular cancers as well as Hodgkin's disease and non-Hodgkin's lymphoma. The side effects are generally gastrointestinal in nature, and include nausea and vomiting, abdominal pain and distension, and constipation or diarrhea. Effects to the bone marrow generally result in a decreased white blood-cell count. Radiation therapy fields over large areas of bone will further reduce blood counts. Radiation delivered to the stomach and intestines will further aggravate nausea and diarrhea.

VP-16 (Etoposide) can be used to treat some types of lung cancer and testicular cancer. Blood count may be lowered, and patients may experience nausea and vomiting. A moderate amount of hair loss is also to be expected. Radiation therapy can further lower the blood count if the treatment fields are large and include extensive areas of bone.

OTHER ANTICANCER SUBSTANCES

The *cortisone* drugs Prednisone and Decadron are sometimes used for breast cancer, multiple myeloma, Hodgkin's disease, and non-Hodgkin's lymphoma because they retard the growth of cancer cells. The drugs are also used to decrease swelling of brain or spinal tissues caused by tumors in these areas. High doses of cortisone medications are effective in treating leukemia and lymphomas because they have a direct destructive effect on the cancer cells and retard their proliferation.

Cortisone drugs may cause weight gain, fluid retention in body tissues, loss of bone mass (osteoporosis), heartburn, ulcers, and increased appetite. (These symptoms are also common when the drug is used to treat conditions other than cancer.) They may also produce a sense of well-being—obviously, a positive side effect.

Hormonal agents are also important chemical treatments commonly administered for breast and prostate cancer, and for cancer of the lining of the uterus. The following three drugs are often used:

EULEXIN (Flutamide). The male hormone testosterone is known to stimulate the growth of prostate cancer. Eulexin is used to block the action of testosterone in the cancer cell, thereby suppressing the hormone's influence. It is used to treat prostate cancers, particularly those that have been spread to bone, causing pain. (Further discussion of these treatments is found in the sections on individual radiation treatment.) Another agent, Lupron (Leuprolide), is combined with Eulexin.

NOLVADEX (Tamoxifen) is a drug used to treat breast cancer. It is most often used to treat postmenopausal women whose cancer has spread from the breast to adjacent lymph nodes. It has been shown to be effective in retarding cancer growth in significant numbers of women. The drug is widely used when it is thought (due to high risk factors) that cancer cells may be circulating through the body, but are not yet detected (adjuvant chemotherapy).

Nolvadex works by blocking the estrogen receptor site on the tumor cell in those breast cancers that are stimulated by estrogen. Its most common side effects are nausea, vomiting, hot flashes, vaginal discharge, and, occasionally, increased bone pain. Radiation to the breast does not aggravate these side effects. Recent reports indicate that some breast cancers may become resistant to Tamoxifen treatment.

MEGACE (Megestrol) is a hormonelike drug whose exact action is unknown; it is used to treat advanced breast, uterine, and prostate cancers. Radiation does not usually aggravate its side effects.

OTHER ISSUES

Because chemotherapeutic drugs and radiation therapy suppress the immune system, drugs that will boost it again are constantly being developed. In addition, these drugs will stimulate the body's own natural defenses against the cancer. Examples of the latter are the interferons and interleukins. A currently used immune system stimulant is Levamisole (ergamisole). It may be prescribed for the treatment of colon cancer.

Radiologists and chemotherapists are partners in your cancer treatment, and every attempt is made to minimize uncomfortable side effects and pain. When we work closely with patients and their families, we can help make periods of treatment as easy as possible while increasing chances for recovery. In the future, I believe we will see more and better combination treatments for cancer.

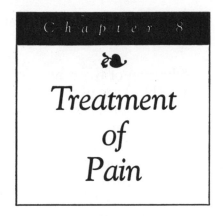

Chapter 8

Treatment
of
Pain

ABOUT ONE-THIRD of all patients undergoing treatment for cancer require medication to control pain. For patients with advanced disease, the figure rises to over two-thirds. As the survival rates for cancer improve, many more patients have been afflicted with pain from the disease. In other words, because of advances in treatment, patients with cancers that were at one time fatal now have their lives extended, and they may experience periodic flare-ups that cause pain.

About 70 percent of patients who experience pain are able to get relief through medications. When medications are combined with radiation therapy and surgical procedures specifically designed to block pain, the remaining 30 percent of patients can be helped. Chemotherapy is as a rule not as effective in reducing pain as radiation therapy and often takes time to do so. However, hormonal therapy for *advanced* breast and prostate cancer is often very effective in treating bone pain when the disease is widespread. Surgery is effective only in specialized situations, such as the relief of intestinal blockage or of pressure on the spinal cord and its nerves caused by the cancer. Radiation therapy is usually the most rapid and effective treatment for relieving pain, particularly pain caused by bone metastases.

WHY IS CANCER PAINFUL?

The origin of most cancer pain is related to tumors causing pressure and destruction of bone. Pain will also occur as the result of

135

nerve compression, infiltration of the cancer in soft tissues and organs, and pressure on or blockage of the gastrointestinal tract. Pain resulting from cancer *treatments* affects only a minority of patients (approximately 10 percent).

Radiation therapy is most effective when used to treat bone pain, and relief is generally accompanied by arrest or eradication of the cancer in the bone under treatment. (X-rays and nuclear bone scans often document this.) In the majority of cancer patients, pain is caused by cancer invading the skeleton or adjacent nerve endings. Pain caused by conditions other than bone destruction due to cancer is not as easily relieved by radiation. For example, cancers causing pressure on nerves are often more effectively treated with cortisone and narcotics.

Pain is strongly influenced by emotions, and people react differently to the same pain stimuli. Some patients are in a distraught psychological state, usually involving fear of disability or death and worry about financial matters, as well as a sense of isolation and loneliness. These emotional concerns will affect the perception of the intensity of the pain among individual patients. Because the brain is capable of producing its own painkillers (endorphins), techniques to stimulate their production can be effective. Meditation, imaging, and biofeedback are examples of these techniques.

In addition, the fear of pain may increase the perception of the pain itself. In other words, a host of physical and emotional factors interplay, and your physician will evaluate all of them when treating you.

PAIN-RELIEF MEDICATIONS

Your physician must consider many factors when prescribing pain medication. First, the *origin* of the pain (bone, muscle, or nerve) must be determined. Each site may require different treatment regimens. Cancer pain that is caused by muscle spasm or swelling of tissues is different from that caused by bone disease. In practical terms, this means that medication that is effective for one kind of pain may be ineffective for another.

Medications may be used alone or in combinations. For example, cortisone medications such as Prednisone or Decadron are particularly effective when used with morphine to relieve severe pain caused by pressure on nerves. The combination is much more effective than using either medication alone. Therefore, it is important that your physician attempt to determine the reason for the pain, not just its location.

When medicating a patient, the physician usually starts with the weakest drugs and then increases a dosage until a satisfactory response occurs. Medications such as aspirin, ibuprofen, and acetaminophen (Tylenol) are frequently used initially. If these fail, the weaker narcotic drugs such as codeine, and oxycodone with aspirin (Percodan) are considered next. The strongest drugs such as morphine, levorphanol (Levo-Dromoran), hydromorphine (Dilaudid), and meperidine (Demerol) are reserved for the most severe pain. The narcotic most commonly used (and the standard for comparison) is morphine. Recently, long-acting oral morphine agents such as M S Contin and Roxanol have become available and have proved very effective. Patients and family members are free from the annoyance and time constraints of injections, as well as the tissue irritation they cause.

When discussing narcotics, it is essential for patients and family members to understand the meaning of the terms *tolerance*, *physical dependency*, and *psychological dependency*. By tolerance, we mean that a particular dosage of pain medication that was satisfactory for a while eventually becomes less effective. In other words, the body has accustomed itself to a level of medication, and therefore its effect is reduced. When this happens, your doctor should not hesitate to increase the dose to make you more comfortable. When pain is severe, medication should be administered around the clock rather than on an "as needed" basis. Although some patients stay on the same dose for long periods of time, other patients reach tolerance more quickly. Doctors know this has happened when patients note that the effect of the medication wears off more quickly, hence the time needed between doses decreases.

When medications must be increased because of tolerance, patients often begin to worry about physical dependency (addiction). They are also concerned about developing a psychological craving for the drug. Most cancer therapists agree that psychological addiction is extremely rare. Patients should not suffer pain because of a fear of dependency, and dosages of narcotics should be adequate to control pain. For the majority of patients, the use of narcotics decreases as radiation therapy successfully reduces pain.

The most common side effects of narcotic medication are constipation, nausea, and oversedation. Your physician will suggest laxatives, stool softeners, and dietary changes that can relieve constipation. Medications to reduce nausea are available and may be useful if the nausea does not gradually disappear on its own. Sedation is an unfortunate side effect, because cancer patients may already have low energy levels and feel fatigued.

Generally, radiation therapists prescribe pain medications, but their knowledge of their use may not be as extensive as that of medical oncologists. We usually leave it to these specialists to fine-tune the use and dosage of narcotic medications. However, radiation therapists are always aware of the medications you are taking and monitor their effectiveness. During the course of radiation therapy, you will be asked about pain, and as it lessens, decisions about reducing medications can be made. Your family physician will also be aware of other conditions that your medical oncologist and radiation therapist should be told about, because these conditions will influence the types of medication used during your treatment.

When all else fails, specialized neurosurgical procedures may be required to block pain. One procedure is to inject chemicals into the nerves, another is to sever the nerve fibers. Surgery may also be used to reduce tumor size and thus relieve pressure on nerve fibers.

Pain is not necessarily a sign of advanced cancer—*curable cancers may cause pain.* It is important for you to remember that pain is not a sign of weakness or something to be ashamed of. When you experience pain or reactions to medications, don't hesitate to talk about what is happening to you. In almost all cases, something can be done to make you more comfortable. For a list of symptoms and their most effective medications, see page 198.

PART 3

Other Issues in Radiation Therapy

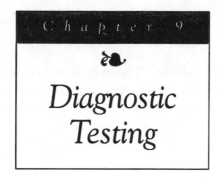

Chapter 9

Diagnostic Testing

WHEN PATIENTS describe symptoms that suggest the presence of cancer, physicians will attempt to locate the possible cancer and then take the necessary steps to either rule out the condition or offer a definitive diagnosis.

Physical examination may reveal a cancer that is apparent to the naked eye. Skin cancers, for example, can be easily seen by a physician trained to recognize them. Cancers of the prostate gland, testicles, rectum, lymph nodes, the female reproductive organs, breast, and the thyroid gland and mouth can often be detected by physical examination. Physicians palpate, or feel, the affected area and determine if an irregularity may be a cancer. Throat and intestinal cancers can be diagnosed with endoscopes, specialized tubes that allow the examiner to view areas within these internal structures. Laboratory tests may provide additional diagnostic information, and some of these tests—the Pap smear, for example—provide a definitive diagnosis of cancer.

Because of their size and location, many other cancers may not be detected without specialized *imaging* examinations. These tests allow physicians to look inside the body. The results of imaging tests are often so suggestive of cancer that a biopsy is performed to confirm or disprove the initial suspicion of cancer.

Test results are used to help plan treatment regimens, monitor progress during treatment, and as part of the follow-up care after treatment is complete. Although some general guidelines exist for treating various cancers, the treatment plan for each patient is individualized. The amount and kind of testing ordered for one person with colon cancer, for example, may not be the same as that recommended for another with the same disease. The person's age, other coexisting conditions, and the stage of the disease will be considered when treatment and follow-up testing are planned.

TYPES OF TESTS

If your primary-care physician believes that a particular type of cancer may be present, he or she will refer you to other specialists who will perform the examinations necessary to confirm the diagnosis. Radiologists perform imaging tests, which include x-rays, nuclear scans, CT scans, ultrasound, and MRI scans. The radiologist determines which test is most able to substantiate or disprove the primary-care physician's initial impression. A *positive* test result means the presence of disease; a *negative* result means that disease is not present or has not been detected.

Obviously, the more tests performed, the more likely it is that a definitive diagnosis will result. However, for many reasons, cost certainly being one of them, radiologists attempt to choose the test that is likely to be the most accurate in the first place, thereby eliminating the need for further testing. The lay person might assume that the most technologically sophisticated—and therefore the most expensive—test may be the best choice. However, this is not always the case. A simple x-ray test may diagnose a particular cancer as accurately as the more complex MRI examination. On the other hand, one MRI scan may be less expensive than a battery of the more simple tests. The radiologist and the other physicians working with you will explain the reasons for choosing a particular test, and I urge you to ask questions about the type of tests being ordered.

The various x-ray tests and other imaging examinations included in this section are also used to diagnose diseases other than cancer. I have described some of the other reasons for these tests so that you will have information about their use.

REVIEW OF TEST RESULTS PRIOR TO RADIATION TREATMENTS

Once a diagnosis of cancer has been established and it is determined that radiation treatment is appropriate, your radiation therapist will plan your course of treatment. Imaging tests used in the diagnostic process are reviewed in order to design the size and shape of the treatment field (portal). The tumor is part of the treatment field, which may also include the usual pathways by which the particular cancer is known to spread. The imaging tests indicate the patterns of spread as well as the depth of the tumor inside the body. Thus, the tests are used both to design the size of the treatment field and to determine the depth of treatment necessary in each individual case.

TESTING DURING TREATMENT

During radiation treatment, physical examinations and imaging tests are necessary to evaluate results. Each person's condition is unique, and there are no standard rules by which physicians determine what tests are needed and when they should be done.

Imaging tests make it possible to determine the effect of radiation on the tumor, thereby allowing the treatment plan to be altered. The treatment portal size may be reduced or reshaped, and the dosage may also be changed. When patients can see that their cancer is improving because of the radiation treatment, they are encouraged by their progress and their spirits lift. Testing may also reassure apprehensive patients that new symptoms are not caused by spreading cancer. For example, when bone pain arises in areas not treated, x-rays or nuclear bone scans may be performed to differentiate, for example, between cancer and arthritis.

Testing is occasionally done to evaluate noncancerous conditions that occur as a result of radiation therapy or have occurred incidental to it. For example, patients may develop gastrointestinal problems that cannot be explained as side effects of the radiation therapy. A GI series or barium enema may be performed to evaluate this separate complaint.

TESTING AFTER COMPLETION OF RADIATION THERAPY

There is significant controversy about the timing and frequency of posttreatment imaging tests. Although guidelines have been established for most cancers, they are arbitrary. These guidelines have been developed as a result of studies that included large numbers of patients with similar cancers. Therefore, they serve as recommendations, but most oncologists continue to individualize each patient's treatment plan and follow-up care.

The results of a physical examination and the patient's symptoms, or lack of them, influence decisions about the type and frequency of testing. Theoretically, a cancer patient could frequently undergo many tests. This approach allows for the earliest possible detection of change in health status. Conversely, frequent tests can demonstrate that no recurring disease exists. However, because of expense and time, risks must be weighed against possible benefits, and a balance must be reached. The type of cancer treated and its stage at the time of its detection will greatly influence decisions about follow-up testing.

When patients are free of their disease, the interval between imaging tests usually lengthens. Actuarial statistics that are used to define cure rates help determine long-term follow-up procedures. For example, a man whose tests reveal no evidence of prostate cancer five years after treatment may be tested less often than he was one year following treatment, because the statistical risk of recurrence decreases with time.

The following tests, briefly described below, are arranged in order of their technological complexity, from what are commonly referred to as low-tech tests to high-tech ones. They include bone x-ray, chest x-ray, barium enema, gastrointestinal examination (GI series), intravenous pyelogram examination (IVP), lymphangiogram, mammogram, myelogram, nuclear scan, ultrasound, computed tomography (CT scan) scanning, and magnetic resonance imaging (MRI scan).

Bone X-Ray

X-rays of the bone are usually performed following an injury in which a resulting fracture is suspected. On x-rays, fractures appear as lines across the bone; when the injury is severe, the break appears as fragments of bone. Bone x-rays are also obtained to evaluate infections and tumors.

Bone x-ray tests are painless, although patients might be in pain because of the injury or condition which prompted the x-rays to be ordered. Most standard bone x-rays include a front view, a side view, and an angled view, called an oblique projection. All of these views are necessary because the overlapping fragment may be aligned so well that the break is revealed only when viewed from a different angle. Smaller but clinically significant fractures are particularly likely to be missed unless multiple projections are obtained. Bone x-rays performed for trauma are highly accurate in detecting an injury.

Bone x-rays are generally not as accurate as nuclear bone scans in revealing *early* signs of infection or tumors. Unlike the sharply defined breaks seen with traumatic fracture, infection and tumors of bone that have progressed past the early stage may appear on x-rays as irregular black holes. (Bone tumors usually are the result of the spread of cancer from distant sites.) These conditions often weaken the bone and cause it to fracture. Cancer spread to bone may also show up as spots of increased bone formation rather than holes (increased whiteness). Both effects may coexist. The beneficial results of radiation therapy and hormone therapy may be seen on the x-ray by the reappearance of normal bone and the healing of fractures.

Chest X-Ray

The "routine" chest x-ray is generally used as a screening tool—that is, to detect diseases for which symptoms have not yet appeared. Lung cancer often fits in this category. Annual chest x-rays may be recommended, particularly for smokers and other high-risk individuals. Naturally a chest x-ray is obtained when symptoms suggest lung or heart problems.

No specific preparation is needed prior to a chest x-ray. At the time the x-ray is taken, the patient is asked to take a deep breath and not exhale until the image is taken, a matter of a few seconds. The air acts as a naturally occurring "contrast agent" to differentiate between structures of varying densities. The lungs are best visualized when fully expanded, which occurs only when one inhales deeply. The chest x-ray is a painless procedure.

The chest x-ray provides an image of the lungs, including the air spaces, the large bronchial tubes, the blood vessels, and the spaces and tissues around the lungs (pleurae). The heart, the major blood vessels and lymph nodes of the center of the chest (mediastinum), the diaphragm (the muscles used for breathing), and the rib cage are also imaged.

Radiologists analyze the lungs (lung fields) for abnormalities, and if present, they evaluate their size, number, and shape. Certain characteristics differentiate cancers from benign diseases. The presence of scattered irregular densities (infiltrates) in the lungs often indicates pneumonia or heart failure. Masses may suggest cancer. In order to arrive at a specific diagnosis, further tests (usually a CT scan and a biopsy) are needed.

The heart is examined for abnormalities in size and shape. Lymph nodes are analyzed to determine if any are enlarged and blood vessels are examined for abnormalities. A chest x-ray will also reveal fluid that has collected in the spaces around the lungs (pleural tissues).

The PA view (posterior anterior projection) is a one-view, frontal chest x-ray. It is usually satisfactory for a routine examination. When physicians desire more information or when symptoms are present, they obtain a two-view chest x-ray that includes a lateral (side) projection of the chest. The more views obtained, the easier it is to precisely localize the position of a suspected abnormality. Thus, when additional views are ordered, this usually indicates the need to further identify an abnormality or clarify its cause.

Although the chest x-ray is quite sensitive for the detection of disease, pulmonary diseases often are *nonspecific* in their presentation. Pneumonias of various causes look like one another, and cancers may sometimes lurk under a pneumonia. An x-ray may reveal nodules, often as small as two millimeters, which are also often nonspecific. Many conditions may cause these nodules to form, and patients may undergo a series of x-rays in order to arrive at a diagnosis based upon the progression of the disease. Comparing recent x-rays with earlier ones helps to determine if changes are of recent origin (indicating acute disease) or have been present for a long time (indicating chronic disease).

A chest x-ray can often allow early detection of abnormalities of the lung coverings (pleurae). Conditions affecting the pleurae are usually manifested by collections of fluid called *effusions*. Most often these pleural effusions are associated with heart failure, but they can also be seen with a variety of other diseases, such as infection or tumors.

Chest x-rays are not as accurate for detecting disease in lymph nodes, because these structures must enlarge a great deal for the change to be detected. The CT scan is much more accurate for their detection. Diseases that cause lymph-node enlargement include lymph-node cancers (lymphomas) and cancer that has spread to lymph nodes from adjacent or distant sites.

The heart shadow is analyzed for its shape and size and the presence of abnormal calcium deposits. If abnormalities are seen, further testing is required to arrive at a specific diagnosis. Ultrasound and nuclear scanning of the heart are more accurate in detecting and specifying cardiac abnormalities.

Gastrointestinal Examination

The upper gastrointestinal series, referred to as a GI series, examines the esophagus (swallowing tube), the stomach, and a portion of the small intestine called the duodenum.

It is common for symptoms from all three areas to mimic one another, and the onset of such symptoms requires that the entire GI series be performed to determine which structure is causing the difficulty. However, other symptoms are specific to the esophagus, and when these occur, only an esophagram is performed. For example, swallowing problems, experienced as lumps or sticking sensations in the throat or chest or a sensation of food coming up from the stomach to the esophagus or throat (regurgitation) are common complaints that may be evaluated by an esophagram. Generally, however, symptoms such as bloating, pain, nausea, and indigestion are evaluated with the entire GI series.

The patient first drinks a barium-sulfate solution. Barium sulfate, the contrast agent, is a fluid that creates greater contrast between the filled organ and the surrounding tissues, enabling abnormalities caused by disease to be identified. Most patients find the barium sulfate palatable, but they experience a sense of fullness as the stomach distends with the drink. The solution fills the esophagus, stomach, and duodenum. Abnormal motion as well as abnormal organ shapes and contours may indicate any of several conditions including inflammation, ulceration (holes in the linings of the organ), and benign and malignant tumors.

Inflammation often causes abnormal motion in the flow of the barium-sulfate solution. Ulcers, which are usually associated with inflammation, are seen in profile as abnormal projections of barium arising from the normal contour of the esophagus, stomach, or duodenum. Cancers tend to form masses, which protrude into the affected structure and alter its shape.

It is necessary to fast before undergoing a GI series. Food particles prevent the complete and even distribution of barium and alter the contour of the gastrointestinal tract, which results in changes that mimic disease. Food particles may also obscure some conditions, particularly ulcers. Fluid intake is also prohibited because it may prevent barium from adequately coating the organs under examination.

During the examination, the radiologist uses fluoroscopy to see the organs in motion. Fluoroscopy is the use of x-rays to create an image of the internal organs and to visualize their motion. Additional x-ray views in different positions usually complete the examination. The position and number of views may be modified by the radiologist depending upon the x-ray findings at the time of the examination.

The amount of barium used and the rate at which it is ingested is modified by what the radiologist sees during the examination. For example, the radiologist may ask the patient to alter the size of the barium "swallows" or to stop drinking at certain points. He or she may also ask the patient to briefly stop breathing while x-ray pictures are being taken of the organs. The entire examination lasts approximately 15 to 20 minutes.

It is common for patients to experience a bloating sensation during or after the examination. This is caused by the barium sulfate. The barium will eventually pass through the entire intestine to the large bowel and out through the feces. Barium will solidify to some extent as it passes through the intestines. Therefore, patients are advised to drink plenty of fluids after the examination is completed. A mild laxative may also be suggested to prevent solidification that can lead to painful bowel movements later in the day.

The GI series is considered fairly accurate in the diagnosis of ulcer diseases and cancers. With the advent of endoscopy, a procedure that uses flexible tubing to allow direct visualization of the stomach and duodenum, diseases can be diagnosed even more accurately. Many patients now undergo endoscopy alone, or after an abnormality has been detected on the GI series, particularly when cancer is suspected. The biopsy may be performed through the endoscope and a diagnosis arrived at directly.

BARIUM ENEMA. Most patients are quite apprehensive about undergoing this examination. Admittedly, the idea of fluid being introduced into the rectum through a tube is unpleasant. However, it is *less* nasty than people usually fear, and while unpleasant, it is a valuable diagnostic tool. The test is performed to detect diseases of the large bowel (large intestine). A barium-sulfate solution is introduced into the bowel through a tube inserted in the rectum. The complete filling of the bowel is monitored by fluoroscopy, the use of x-rays to create an image of internal organs and to visualize their motion. Diverticulae (saclike protrusions), inflammatory disease (colitis), polyps (mushroomlike growths), and cancers can be detected with a barium enema. This test is also used to determine the effects of abnormalities of adjacent organs on the bowel.

Large-bowel disease may include one or more of the following common symptoms: rectal bleeding; cramping; steady or intermittent abdominal pain; and changes in normal bowel habits, such as diarrhea, constipation, or alternating conditions of each. When infection is present, fever may accompany the bowel symptoms; if bleeding is prolonged or extensive, anemia will result.

The saclike protrusions from the bowel, called diverticulae, normally occur with advancing age and appear to be caused by weakness of the bowel walls, thus allowing these protrusions to form. The condition is called diverticulosis. If the diverticulae become infected, this very painful disease is called diverticulitis. During the examination, barium collects in these diverticulae, and they appear like grapes on a vine. Since inflammatory diseases generally cause the lining of the intestine (mucosa) to swell and or tear (ulcerate), the barium will be displaced by swelling or deposited in the ulcers. These swellings and deposits are fairly well visualized on the barium-enema test.

Polyps, mushroomlike growths, may be benign (noncancerous) or malignant (cancerous). Larger polyps are more likely to be malignant than smaller ones, and they sometimes cause rectal bleeding. Cancers can appear as polyps on the barium enema. Large, cancerous irregularities of the bowel wall may lead to obstruction.

The bowel must be clean and free of all fecal material. At the time of the testing, all radiological facilities provide instructions to accomplish this, and dietary restrictions designed to decrease bulk and increase liquidity are essential. Laxatives and cleansing enemas supplement the diet, which must be followed the day before the test.

A tube is inserted in the rectum in order to administer the barium enema. Technicians have been trained to do this gently, and it is a relatively painless event. If you lie on your side and breath deeply, your body will tend to relax during the insertion. A small balloon attached to the tube is inflated in the rectum. This prevents the barium from leaking back onto the table during the enema, and it causes a slight sensation of pressure in the rectum.

I advise all my patients to lie on their stomach (prone) during the examination. This is contrary to the standard practice of having patients lie supine. My technique allows the bowel to be well visualized and also allows the barium to be accepted more easily by the lower bowel, in that it takes advantage of normal anatomic curves. This technique also decreases the sensation of urgency, namely the need to evacuate the barium during the examination.

Barium acts as a contrast agent, highlighting the bowel by making it more visible against the background of the non-barium-filled organs. Thus irregularities in the contour and shape of the bowel and "filling defects" are readily viewed. While there are different techniques to performing a barium enema, my routine follows.

While the bowel is filled with barium, the radiologist takes pictures of the normal or abnormal findings using the fluoroscope. You may then be asked to evacuate the barium in the bathroom, or it may be drained back into the bag it came from. Air is then introduced into the bowel through a special connection in the original tubing or through insertion of another tube. The air acts as contrast material and, in my opinion, adds to the accuracy of the examination. However, this portion of the test is often accompanied by bloating and cramping due to bowel stretching and distension.

Following the fluoroscopic portion of the test, a technician completes the examination by taking additional standard views under the radiologist's supervision. The air-contrast part of the examination may add another three to five views. The test takes about 30 minutes.

The barium enema is very accurate in detecting diverticulae, but inflammatory diseases usually are more advanced before being revealed on x-rays. Accuracy in detecting polyps depends on how thoroughly the bowel is cleansed. Adding air contrast helps in the accuracy of detection, an important factor because cancerous polyps are not uncommon. The barium enema readily detects most large-bowel cancers, especially those causing irregularities in the contour of the bowel.

Direct visualization techniques using flexible tubes (colonoscopy) are often used as a substitute to barium enemas. Colonoscopy is performed by inserting a flexible tube into the colon, which allows the physician to view the inside of this internal structure. The procedure may be limited to visualizing the left portion of the colon (where most of the cancers arise), or the entire colon, both left and right sides. This test is used to further examine the bowel (1) if the barium enema is interpreted as "negative" (normal) and symptoms warrant further investigation; (2) to confirm or further investigate definite abnormalities seen on barium enema; (3) to take a tissue sample in a diseased area that was seen on barium enema (biopsy); (4) to clarify suspicious changes on barium enema which make the diagnosis uncertain.

Much controversy exists on the merits of colonoscopy as a substitute for the barium enema. My opinion, shared by many radiologists, is that a well-performed barium enema is a good initial examination. In addition, diseases may be missed with colonoscopy. Nevertheless, colonoscopy is a highly accurate examination and involves no radiation. Following treatment for colon cancer, patients must undergo periodic barium-enema, colonoscopy examinations to see if their disease is cured or recurring.

After effects of the barium enema (and colonoscopy) include bloating and cramping, generally from the inserted air. I recommend resting after the examination if possible, because you will be passing air and residual barium periodically for the next few hours. For people with chronic constipation and who tend to have a "sluggish bowel," a mild laxative or a gentle enema will help evacuate the barium so that it will not solidify and cause additional problems.

SMALL-BOWEL SERIES. This test may be performed by itself or as part of the GI series, depending upon symptoms.

As with the GI series, the most common reasons for the examination are to detect inflammatory diseases (ileitis) and cancers. It is also used to determine if an obstruction of the small bowel is present. Patients undergoing radiation therapy to the abdomen or pelvis occasionally require this examination if the side effects are unusually severe and suggest inflammation or obstruction.

Although they can occur, tumors are uncommon in the small intestine. Occasionally, rare conditions caused by various parasites can be detected by the small-bowel study. Certain disease states causing impaired absorption (malabsorption) are also evaluated by the use of this test.

The small-bowel series is a time-consuming examination (an average of two hours) because approximately 20 to 25 feet of intestine must be filled with barium and examined. However, you will not be in the examining room for the entire time. The examination is usually performed at half-hour intervals, and the test is completed when the entire small bowel has been filled. Examinations longer than two to three hours generally indicate a disease process has been identified, because an abnormality will commonly delay the normal passage of barium. Fluoroscopy may be added, depending upon the condition identified.

You will be asked to swallow two to three eight-ounce cups of barium, since that amount is necessary to entirely fill the small intestine.

Intravenous Pyelogram Examination (IVP)

Commonly known as the IVP (intravenous pyelogram), this is a test of kidney function as well as an evaluation of the size and shape of the urinary system. It is a painless examination and is performed under the supervision of a radiologist, who determines the time sequence and appropriate views.

Infection of the kidneys may cause pain in the small of the back (flank pain). Frequency (increased urination), urgency (the sensation of needing to urinate even when the bladder is empty), and burning sensations are common complaints related to bladder infection. Radiation can cause similar symptoms.

A kidney stone lodged in one of the ureters may result in obstruction of the urinary tract. The ureters, one on each side, constitute the major collecting system of the urinary tract. They serve as drainage pipes leading out of the kidneys to the bladder. Obstruction of the ureters may also occur due to tumors of the kidneys.

In males, a frequent cause of bladder obstruction is benign (noncancerous) enlargement of the prostate gland. The gland lies at the bladder outlet. Cancer in the prostate gland may cause obstruction in the bladder and ureters. In females, benign or malignant tumors of the uterus and ovaries may cause obstruction of the ureters.

Depending on the location, obstruction causes a backup situation similar to clogged plumbing. This results in a dilatation (widening) of the system behind the obstruction. Obstruction of the ureters may be so severe as to shut down kidney function and prevent the contrast material used in the IVP from being seen. The IVP is an essential test when blockage is suspected.

Blood in the urine may be caused by an infection, an obstruction caused by stones, or by tumors. Infection will cause abnormal size and shape of the ureters and may, in advanced stages, alter the size and shape of the kidneys. Tumors will also alter the size and shape of the involved organs, often causing irregularities in the contour of those organs.

The contrast agent used in the IVP is an organic iodine compound. It is injected into a vein in the arm and travels through the bloodstream directly to the kidneys, then passes through the kidneys and the ureters. From the ureters, the contrast agent then empties into the bladder. The fluid appears white on an x-ray, contrasting with the grayish and black appearance of surrounding organs, and thus provides a picture of the kidneys, the ureters, and the bladder. The amount of this clear, colorless fluid injected varies according to the patient's weight. Don't be intimidated by the large syringe required. The size of the syringe has nothing to do with the small gauge of the needle used to puncture the vein.

Before the contrast agent is injected, an ordinary x-ray of the abdomen is obtained. Occasionally, a specialized x-ray of the kidneys—called a tomogram—is added. This x-ray device makes a "slice" of the kidney, focusing on a layer that is usually a quarter of an inch thick. By obtaining both of these pictures, calcified stones in the kidneys and ureters can be detected.

The injection should be painless once the needle punctures the skin and enters the vein. If the pain persists during the injection, do not be reluctant to call this to the doctor's or nurse's attention. Persistent pain indicates that the dye is leaking outside the vein and calls for the needle to be repositioned. It is normal to feel flushing and heat, because the dye dilates the blood vessels. You also may experience nausea and a metallic taste sensation.

Although rare, moderate to severe allergic reactions may occur within one to three minutes after the beginning of the injection; more mild reactions appear in the first 10 minutes. Therefore, if any symptoms other than those described above occur, it is important that you call this to the attention of the physician or nurse attending to you. Those attending to you can administer special drugs to counter the allergic reactions. (Physicians and nurses will almost always ask your allergic history before administering an injection. Should they overlook this question, volunteer any information you believe is relevant *before* receiving the injection. Severe allergic histories will occasionally require cancellation of the test.) Although they are very expensive, the newer "nonionic" contrast agents have markedly reduced allergic reactions.

Should they occur, most allergic reactions involve moderate appearance of hives, itching, nasal stuffiness, and tearing. The symptoms promptly clear after the injection of a mild antihistamine. Severe allergies are medical emergencies. In the great majority of cases the examination proceeds smoothly.

The IVP examination is the best test for detecting obstruction from many causes. However, it is somewhat less accurate for imaging tumors of the bladder and kidneys. Therefore, a CT scan or an ultrasound examination may be used in addition to the IVP.

The IVP examination is of only moderate value for detecting sources of bleeding unless stones, kidney tumors, bladder tumors, or prostate-gland enlargement are identified.

Infectious diseases must be quite advanced to alter the x-ray appearance of the kidneys and the ureters. Therefore, infections are not easily detected on the IVP unless they are moderately advanced. Since high blood pressure can be caused by chronic kidney disease, the IVP may be useful in demonstrating small, poorly functioning kidneys. (Most cases of high blood pressure, however, are not caused by kidney disease.) An enlarged prostate gland is easily identified by its pressure on the adjacent bladder.

As mentioned previously, the radiologist closely monitors the IVP during its performance. If the test is normal, expect a 45-minute to one-hour examination time. This may include a film taken after voiding in order to test bladder function, particularly in males with enlargement of the prostate gland. If disease is detected, additional appropriate views are obtained and the examination may last longer.

Lymphangiogram

The lymphangiogram is an infrequently performed test used in the diagnosis of some lymph-node cancers. There are thousands of lymph nodes widely distributed throughout the body, which act as biological filters. When a lymphangiogram is used, it is generally for the purpose of examining the lymph nodes in the pelvic and abdominal areas.

The test requires that an x-ray fluid known as a contrast agent or dye be injected into the lymph system. It is usually injected into a lymph vessel on the top of the foot. (A local anesthetic is applied to the skin to lessen the discomfort caused by the placement of the needle.) This part of the test takes approximately 30 minutes to perform and is a very painstaking procedure.

The lymph vessels are filled with dye, and over a period of several hours, x-rays are obtained to examine the lymph nodes and their connecting vessels. The lymph-node groups in the pelvis and the abdomen gradually fill with dye, and their size, shape, and structure can be evaluated. Depending on the type of cancer suspected, an x-ray diagnosis of cancer can be made with some accuracy. The patient is usually lying down for the initial 30 minutes of the examination, and then may leave the examining room and is directed by the radiologist to return some hours later for additional x-rays.

The lymphangiogram may be particularly useful in patients with Hodgkin's disease, prostate cancer, and testicular cancer. By imaging abnormal lymph nodes, the radiation therapist can correctly plan treatment to include all affected areas. However, a normal result does not necessarily mean the disease is not present.

Occasionally, abnormal lymph nodes detected on the lymphangiogram require surgical exploration to confirm the presence of the suspected cancer.

The dye remains in the lymph nodes for months and sometimes years, allowing the radiation therapist to plan the lymph-node treatments at any time. The dye has no adverse effects on the patient. In addition, as treatment progresses, further x-rays can be obtained to determine if the lymph nodes are improving in their appearance, thereby indicating that the cancer is being eradicated.

Mammogram

A mammogram is an x-ray examination of the breast, and is usually done for the purpose of detecting or excluding the presence of cancer. Although this relatively painless procedure has been available for more than 20 years, it has become accepted as a routine screening procedure only in the past decade.

There are two major reasons for the increasing number of mammograms performed annually. One is the marked improvement in the efficiency and safety of the equipment used to perform the test. In addition, technical innovations in x-ray film quality have allowed for improved diagnostic accuracy along with significantly reduced radiation dosage.

The American Cancer Society has strongly endorsed the use of mammography for early breast-cancer detection. It bases its recommendations on the results of extensive studies in which early detection has been fairly conclusively shown to reduce breast-cancer mortality. The Breast Cancer Detection Demonstration Project, begun in 1973 and concluded in 1981, involved 26 university hospital centers and more than 280,000 women. I was involved in this study and served as assistant director of the New Jersey project at the New Jersey College of Medicine and Dentistry. This long-term project revealed that for women over age 50, yearly mammograms lowered the breast-cancer death rate by approximately 30 percent. Because the incidence of breast cancer rises with increasing age, particularly age 50, the results of this study are encouraging.

There are two major reasons for performing mammography. One is for the purpose of screening, and the second is to evaluate a lumpy or painful breast felt by the woman during self-examination or by the physician during an office visit.

The screening mammogram is used to detect diseases not revealed by manual examination. Thus, screening is an important use of mammography because many cancers are discovered while still small and at an early stage in the progression of the disease. In its early stages, breast cancer is highly curable.

The previously mentioned Breast Cancer Detection Demonstration Project produced significant figures in support of using mammography as a tool for early detection. The data showed 88.9 percent of the 3,557 breast cancers discovered by the project were found by mammography, compared to 56 percent by physical examination. Almost 42 percent of the cancers were discovered by mammography alone when physical examination was normal.

Mammography when performed for lumps or thickening in the breast may reveal, in decreasing order of frequency, the presence of inflammation, noncancerous masses, or cancer. The inflammation referred to is usually called fibrocystic disease or fibrocystic condition. These are general terms used to describe a condition consisting of overgrowth of the cells lining the mammary ducts, the milk-producing channels. This condition is often associated with scarring (fibrosis) of the breast tissue and fluid collections called cysts—thus, the term *fibrocystic*.

Cysts appear as round, smooth-bordered densities. Thickening of ducts and scarring reveal themselves as coarse or fine linear densities. Clumps of large, coarse calcium deposits caused by this condition are easily seen on the mammogram. Radiologists are able to recognize the patterns of fibrocystic disease and differentiate these from other breast conditions.

Women with fibrocystic disease may or may not experience pain. Some premenopausal women report discomfort only prior to the onset of menstruation, while others speak of breast tenderness or unusual sensitivity throughout their cycles. Yellow or greenish discharge from the nipple may also occur.

Breast cancers have their own specific pattern. On an x-ray, they are generally seen as irregularly shaped masses. Often the edges of the masses have linear strands much like the picture of sun rays. In about 50 percent of the cancers, the mammogram will reveal small particles of calcium produced by the tumor. Called microcalcifications, they help confirm the diagnosis. On occasion cancers are detected solely by the presence of these microcalcifications because no mass is evident. In these cases, the cancer is rarely discovered on physical examination by the patient or her doctor since the calcium deposits are too small to be felt. Cancers the size of the head of a pin are routinely detected with modern mammographic technique. In order to help the surgeon biopsy and confirm a suspected cancer that can't be felt, the radiologist will place a needle in the breast (needle localization) to guide the surgeon to the proper spot.

The mammogram also helps physicians evaluate the effects of the cancer on the adjacent breast tissue, the lymph nodes, and the skin. This helps physicians differentiate between the early stage of the disease and the more advanced cancers.

The value of the mammogram can be seen more clearly when we consider that in the early stage, breast cancer can't be felt. Even when somewhat larger, the masses may not be felt unless they happen to be close to the surface of the breast or when the breast is small. In other words, a woman with a small breast may feel a mass if it is close to the surface, while the exact same size cancer may not be manually detected if it is located deep in a large breast.

Generally, cancers feel firm to the touch and are not painful when examined either by the woman herself or a physician. They also have a consistency we sometimes describe as pebbled. This differentiates a cancerous mass from the more rubbery consistency of fibrocystic lumps and thickenings. When the cancers are larger, they become isolated firm areas that may or may not be painful. Puckering and ulceration of the overlying skin are also associated with larger cancers. In addition, bloody discharge from the nipple may occur.

Because cancer and fibrocystic disease can coexist, a mammogram may help distinguish the two conditions. When only physical examination is done, cancer and fibrocystic disease can be mistaken for one another because symptoms sometimes mimic one another. Also it is not uncommon for a fibrocystic mass to lie next to a cancer. This prevents the examining fingers from distinguishing the lethal lesion from its innocent neighbor.

The American Cancer Society has established guidelines for mammography for women who are asymptomatic, meaning that no breast problems are apparent.

Briefly they are:

1. Women between 35 and 40 should have a baseline mammogram. A baseline mammogram is a picture of the breast when it is presumed to be free of any disease. This mammogram can be used for comparison at a later date when other mammograms are taken. Early but significant abnormalities can often be detected by comparison of the mammogram baseline with later mammograms.

2. Asymptomatic women 40 to 49 should have a mammography every one to two years. Women over 50 should have a mammogram once a year.

3. Women with a personal or family history of breast cancer should talk with their physicians about the need for more frequent mammograms. They should also discuss beginning periodic mammograms before age 50.

Remember, the above guidelines apply to those women who do not have symptoms. The American Cancer Society goes on to state: "Since the symptomatic woman with a dominant mass or persistent discomfort, nipple discharge, or other symptoms may have breast cancer, *all* such women should have a thorough breast examination including mammography and any other diagnostic study to determine if cancer is present."

Mammography does not require any special preparation except the avoidance of deodorants and powders, which may contain particles that mimic abnormal calcifications on the mammogram. Two views of the breast are generally obtained. In the first, the women is seated and the x-ray beam traverses from top to bottom, the cranial-caudal view. The second is a side view, with the x-ray beam traversing from one side of the breast to the other. In this lateral view the woman may be seated or lying down, depending on the type of x-ray equipment used.

Additional views of the breast may be needed if there is a question about the diagnosis or if the entire breast tissue cannot be seen in the standard two views. However, the two-view examination is usually adequate.

Mammography generally lasts three to five minutes. The breast is slightly compressed for the examination by a plastic plate, to make the thickness of the breast tissue as uniform as possible and thus enhance photographic quality. This compression causes moderate discomfort. If breasts are very painful to begin with, this compression may seem unpleasant although not lasting more than the "set-up time" of approximately 30 seconds.

Many radiologists prefer that premenopausal women undergo mammography during the first two weeks of their menstrual cycles, particularly if a woman has an extensive fibrocystic condition to begin with. Densities seen on the mammogram due to fibrocystic disease may obscure the outlines of a cancerous lesion. Because the breasts tend to be less sensitive during the first two weeks of the hormonal cycle, the previously described compression will not seem quite as severe.

I like to review the mammogram immediately after it is obtained to determine technical adequacy and the need for further views. If the diagnosis is inconclusive, I will physically examine the patient's breasts.

The accuracy rate of the mammogram is about 95 percent for the detection of cancer. In about five percent of cases the initial diagnosis is incorrect. For example, the radiologist may interpret a noncancerous (benign) abnormality as a cancer. When a benign abnormality is diagnosed as cancer, we call this a *false positive* interpretation. Conversely, calling a cancerous abnormality benign is a *false negative* interpretation. Thus, a radiologist can misinterpret a mammogram since benign and malignant lesions can mimic one another.

Erroneous mammographic diagnosis may occur because a minority of cancers are simply not imaged, meaning that they don't appear on the x-ray. This usually has to do with the density of the surrounding breast tissues adjacent to the cancer. Specifically, the borders of the cancer may blend with the surrounding normal tissues and obscure the tumor. When the breast tissue on the mammogram is especially dense and there is a clinical suspicion of cancer, a biopsy is mandatory even if the mammogram is interpreted as normal. Obviously, it is best to err on the side of caution.

Cysts are usually benign, but they can occasionally harbor a cancer. If there is just one cyst, or if a cyst is particularly large, it will be drained with a needle, a procedure known as aspiration. The fluid content is analyzed for the possible presence of cancerous cells. Yellowish fluid usually is not associated with cancers, but bloody fluid may be associated with cancer. When many are present, the larger cysts are usually aspirated. A repeat mammogram is then often performed after several months to reevaluate the breast. A cyst requiring more than two or three drainages over a short period of time is usually surgically removed since it may contain a cancer.

Women who have had a mastectomy should undergo periodic screening mammographies of the opposite breast since there is an increased likelihood of cancer in that breast. Similarly, women who have undergone a lumpectomy (see chapter 5) should have periodic mammograms to make sure the cancer does not recur in the remaining breast tissue or the opposite breast.

Few women submit to mammography without some apprehension and in some cases I've seen, intense fear. The women I've talked with who have serious reservations about mammography are usually afraid that the test itself will increase their chances of developing breast cancer. However, with the current low-dosage examination, this possibility is minimal when compared to the benefits of early detection.

Women *most* at risk for breast cancer, those over the age of 50, are *least* likely to be affected adversely by repeated radiation exposures to the breast. Conversely, women between the ages of 20 and 30, those with breast tissue more sensitive to adverse radiation effects, rarely need to undergo periodic mammography unless signs of serious breast disease are present.

The low dosage used in current mammography is the result of greatly improved photographic technology and x-ray tube construction in recent years. Radiologists have become increasingly sensitive to the importance of minimizing the number of exposures to mammography, and technicians have become more knowledgeable in the techniques of this examination. Actually, the current dosages are even *less* than those recommended by the National Cancer Institute. As new technology is developed, further reduction in radiation dosages will likely occur. I suggest that women focus on the examination's life-saving potential, because such large numbers of women will at some time in their lives be diagnosed as having breast cancer.

Myelogram

The myelogram is performed less frequently than in the past, because it has been greatly replaced by the CT and MRI scans. Nevertheless myelography remains a good means of detecting obstruction to the flow of spinal fluid caused by the spread of cancer from a distant site.

The myelogram evaluates the spinal canal and the spinal cord, enclosed by the bony spine (vertebrae) and bathed in spinal fluid. When CT and MRI scans are not available, this test is used to detect herniated (ruptured) discs, which are protrusions of the tissue between the vertebrae. These protrusions can cause pressure on the spinal cord or its nerve roots. The test is also used to detect tumors, which have either originated in the spine or have spread from a distant site. The myelogram is also useful in evaluating trauma and infection. However, where the technology is available, CT and MRI scans have largely replaced the myelogram for the above purposes.

The spinal canal is filled with a contrast agent and analyzed for the following patterns: (1) partial or total blockages; (2) changes in contour—that is, defects and irregularities in the shape of the contrast filled space; (3) changes in the size of the spinal canal; (4) changes in the appearance of the spinal cord.

This procedure can be uncomfortable and even painful, because the patient's symptoms are often debilitating to begin with. A mild sedative is usually administered before the examination to lessen discomfort and anxiety. A local anesthetic is injected into the skin, and a needle is then inserted into the spinal canal. This procedure is often accompanied by fluoroscopic observation to check the needle position. (Fluoroscopy involves the use of x-rays to visualize internal procedures.) The contrast agent is then injected into the spinal canal. The newer contrast agents are iodinated water-soluble organic compounds that mix with the spinal fluid and are readily absorbed and excreted by the body. The amount of contrast agent injected is determined by the size of the spinal canal and by the disease process being evaluated. The needle is removed after the injection.

X-ray pictures are obtained of the patient in different positions, according to the findings visualized. The table will be tilted to allow the contrast agent to flow to different parts of the spinal canal.

The contrast agents used can be irritating to the nervous system, and they have the potential to cause seizures. To lessen this possibility, the patient may be given the drug, usually phenobarbital for several days prior to the test. Patients are encouraged to drink plenty of fluids before and after the examination so that the contrast agent will be rapidly eliminated by the kidneys.

Patients will feel a sharp pain when the local anesthetic is applied to the skin of the back. The next sensation is the momentary sharp pain of the needle piercing the cover of the spinal canal. From that point on, the insertion of the fluid is painless. Similarly, the various maneuvers performed for the test are painless.

Patients may experience headaches, nausea and vomiting, and muscle pains after the test. In order to prevent the contrast agent from flowing to the brain and causing severe headaches, it is important to keep the head raised for a day following the test. These after effects may begin immediately or a few hours after the test, and they may last up to 72 hours.

The myelogram is an accurate test to evaluate the effects of a herniated disc on the spinal canal and the nerve roots. It is especially accurate in revealing blockages. In most technologically sophisticated facilities, a myelogram may be performed a few hours prior to a CT scan as an ancillary test. The contrast-filled spinal canal can be well visualized on the CT scan, which may help in arriving at a diagnosis in difficult cases.

Nuclear Scanning

Nuclear scanning involves the imaging of organs (such as the liver, bones, heart, or lungs) that have been made to temporarily emit x-rays (gamma rays). This is effected by swallowing or injecting radioactive substances (isotopes). The image that results is called a scan. Over the past 25 years, newer and safer isotopes have been developed, resulting in decreased radiation dosage while increasing the accuracy of the examination.

Biochemists have devised ways to combine certain chemicals with these isotopes in a process called labeling, so that the scanning agents seek out the particular organ (target organ) to be examined. For example, combining the technetium-99 isotope with sulfur colloid will trap most of the isotope in certain liver cells. By using a device that can detect and record the radioactivity emitted from the liver, an image of the liver can be transcribed to x-ray film as a permanent record. When we combine the same technetium-99 isotope with methylene diphosphonate, the isotope seeks bone rather than liver.

Various combinations of chemical substances labeled with different isotopes allow the body organs to be visualized and disease states identified. Other individual isotopes seek out organs by virtue of the organ's inherent biological activity. For example, since the thyroid gland is involved in iodine storage, swallowing radioactive iodine will image this gland.

Once the scanning agent has been injected or ingested, it travels through the bloodstream where it reaches the target organ. This organ gradually accumulates radioactivity, over a period of time. The rate of accumulation depends upon the isotope used and the biological properties of the particular organ. It is for this reason that there is an interval of several hours between the administration of the agent and the performance of the test.

When the isotope has accumulated, the patient lies or sits, depending on the test, in front of an instrument that detects the radioactivity. This instrument is called a gamma camera, and it never touches the patient at any point during this painless test. The camera is able to detect and "collect" the gamma rays emitted from the target organ. This process is recorded on a video monitor by the nuclear-medicine technician. When enough activity has been recorded to obtain an accurate image, this is transferred onto x-ray film for the radiologist to interpret.

Few of these tests involve side effects or aftereffects from the isotopes. However, since most isotopes are excreted in human milk, a nursing mother should substitute formula feedings for a period of time suggested by her physician.

The following types of nuclear scanning tests are listed alphabetically.

BONE SCAN. The bone scan is the most frequently performed isotope scan for diagnosing cancer. The procedure begins when a technetium-labeled phosphorus-containing scanning agent is injected into an arm vein.

An interval of approximately two hours follows to allow the radioactivity to collect in the skeleton. Since the body rids itself of the isotope through the kidneys and bladder, it is a good idea to force fluid intake and to void often to rid the body of unnecessary radioactivity in the kidneys and bladder. There is no physical sensation associated with the test.

The bone-scan image visualizes the entire skeleton, which is represented as a series of fine black dots with excellent definition so as to show each vertebra, rib, and so on. A *positive* (abnormal) scan is usually seen as an area of increased blackness in a particular bone or group of bones. This increased blackness is a result of increased disease activity in those areas. On occasion a decrease in blackness will likewise indicate an abnormality.

The bone scan is extremely useful for detecting injury. Even though conventional x-rays are very accurate, there are many situations in which the x-ray results are negative (normal) or equivocal. The bone scan, however, may often be positive earlier than the x-ray.

Another value of the bone scan in trauma is to determine the age of the injury. For example, a patient may complain of back pain and x-rays reveal a fractured vertebra; however, the fracture may have been present for years. The bone scan may indicate if the injury is acute or old. With infections or arthritis the bone scan will often reveal the abnormality before the conditions appear on an x-ray.

Bone scanning is of greatest value and most often performed for the detection of metastatic cancer, that is, cancer that has spread from a distant site. The bone scan provides information that reveals the extent of the disease involving one or a group of bones. This is of great help in staging the cancer, as well as planning the location and extent of treatment. It is also of great use in assessing the results of radiation therapy or chemotherapy, because abnormal areas may revert to normal after treatment. Although almost any cancer can spread to the bone, the most common cancers to be evaluated are those originating in the lung, breast, and the prostate gland.

Although the scan is very sensitive in detecting bone disease, it is *nonspecific*. Arthritis, infection, fractures, and cancer may all look the same. Thus, x-rays of the affected bones are often obtained to assist in differentiating these conditions. The patient's history together with the x-rays then clarifies the situation. Follow-up bone scans are extremely important. A comparison will be made with the initial scan, allowing the radiologist to perceive small but *significant* changes.

WHOLE-BODY SCAN (GALLIUM SCANNING). Whole-body scanning is used to search for a hidden source of infection, to evaluate lymph nodes for the presence of cancer (primarily lymphoma), and to evaluate suspected bone infection when the routine bone scan is negative.

The radioisotope gallium-67 is injected intravenously into the bloodstream, and images are usually obtained daily over the next 72 hours. There is no physical sensation associated with this test. Diseases are pictured as regions of increased blackness. Thus, an abscess and a tumor will look identical, both showing up as areas of blackness against the lighter background of various body organs.

Gallium scanning is currently used less frequently than in the past because CT scanning is accurate for detecting hidden cancers and infections. However, when CT scans are equivocal or considered negative, this scanning may resolve the issue when a tumor or an infection is considered likely. Nowadays, gallium scanning is most often ordered when more information is needed to confirm a diagnosis.

LIVER SCAN. The radioactive substance used in a liver scan is technetium-99, labeled sulfur colloid. After an intravenous injection of the agent, imaging is immediately performed in multiple projections in order to visualize all the surfaces of the liver. The scanning is a painless procedure.

The primary reason a liver scan is performed is to detect metastatic cancer, although in facilities with high technologies available, the CT scan has largely replaced the liver nuclear scan for this diagnostic purpose. The liver scan is also used to evaluate the liver for cirrhosis, an inflammation often associated with alcoholism.

The liver is imaged as a series of fine black dots that reveal the shape, size, and position of the organ in the abdominal cavity. Tumors and other abnormal masses are usually detected as areas of absent radioactivity ("defects"). The isotope also travels to the adjacent spleen. Cirrhosis affecting the liver will often also affect the spleen. The sensitivity of the scan to detect disease depends on the size and location of the abnormality.

LUNG SCAN (PULMONARY SCAN). Nuclear imaging of the lung is primarily used to evaluate blood clots (emboli). These clots may form as the result of inflammation in distal veins, usually in the legs (phlebitis); if dislodged from the vein they may travel to the lungs. Abdominal, pelvic, and hip surgery may cause clots to form in the veins. These clots may then travel to the lungs. Occasionally, cancers may predispose a patient to the formation of clots. However, blood clots may also form in the lungs for no obvious reason. The scan is also used to evaluate lung function in patients with lung cancer, emphysema, and other chronic pulmonary diseases where some obstruction of the airway or blood flow may be present.

When feasible, two isotope tests are performed at the same sitting. One test evaluates the blood flow through the lungs and is called the *perfusion scan*. This is accomplished by intravenous injection of technetium-99-labeled particles (macroaggregates). These particles lodge in the small vessels of the lungs. However, the particles are not deposited where clots occur because they act as barriers. These defects can often be observed only by obtaining multiple views of the lungs.

The second test, called the *ventilation scan*, uses a different isotope and evaluates how clear the bronchial airways are. Abnormal ventilation scans are common in patients with emphysema, asthma, and obstruction caused by cancer.

The ventilation scan is performed by inhaling a radioactive gas called xenon-133, which provides fairly accurate information about the condition of the bronchial airways. A bag is filled with the isotope and the patient breathes the aerosol directly, and multiple views of the lungs are obtained.

The ventilation and perfusion scans are often performed one after the other and reviewed simultaneously to reach a definitive diagnosis. They are painless and accurate procedures.

Ultrasound

No radiation is involved in an ultrasound examination. It is an important diagnostic test with no known hazards.

Using a device called a transducer, inaudible high-frequency sound waves are beamed through solid and fluid-filled structures of the body. The echoes bounce off the structures and are returned and collected by the transducer, which is in contact with the patient's body. The series of sound signals are processed electronically, and a display of the anatomical sound image is made on a screen. These images are then transferred to x-ray film for a permanent record. The images formed are anatomical representations of the body organs and disease processes.

Modern ultrasound scanners use so-called "real time" technology, meaning that the pictures analyze not only structures, but their motion as well. This is analogous to the fluoroscopic examination except here sound waves are used, rather than x-rays, to obtain the images.

Normal organs and their tissues reveal specific ultrasound patterns; conversely, diseases have their own characteristic echo patterns.

The ultrasound technician beams the sound waves and collects these echoes with the transducer. A jelly substance is applied to the transducer and the skin to act as a contact so that air does not form a barrier to the sound waves. The pictures obtained are sections or slices (tomographic images) of the area examined. Thus, multiple images must be acquired in order to image the entire organ.

Patients are encouraged to drink plenty of fluid prior to an examination of the pelvis in order to have a full bladder at the time of the ultrasound examination, because sound waves travel best through fluid. A fasting state is necessary for gallbladder ultrasound because food will contract the organ and prevent it from being accurately evaluated. An ultrasound test is painless. A patient will feel moderate pressure as the technician passes the transducer over the skin.

The following ultrasound tests are listed alphabetically.

GYNECOLOGICAL ULTRASONOGRAPHY. Noncancerous and cancerous ovarian and uterine masses are best examined with ultrasound because it is highly accurate for detecting their size, location, and appearance, meaning whether they are solid or fluid-filled. Abnormal fluid around these organs will also be clearly seen. However, the test's specificity, meaning the ability to make a definitive diagnosis, is limited because many infectious and cancerous conditions look the same on ultrasound. Thus, a benign cyst of the ovary may look exactly like an infected cyst caused by pelvic inflammatory disease. Similar abnormalities may be seen with cancers. In order to make the examination more *specific*, the physical examination and the patient's history are extremely important. Follow-up ultrasound examinations may also clarify the diagnosis by showing the evolution of the disease process.

On occasion, CT scans or a laparoscopy, a surgical procedure which allows direct visualization of the gynecologic organs, may be required. CT scans are generally used to evaluate malignant changes and their spread to adjacent pelvic tissues and distant organs. Ultrasound is often used as a screening test, followed by CT scan to obtain a more accurate diagnosis. Because ultrasound does not involve the use of radiation, it is an ideal test for women of childbearing age.

Several hours before the test, the woman will be asked to drink about a quart of water in order to fill the bladder, thus allowing the ultrasound beam to better travel through the body. The woman will lie on the examination couch in a comfortable position. The test itself does not cause any pain, and the only sensation is the pressure of the transducer passing over the skin. The test lasts approximately 15 minutes.

KIDNEY ULTRASONOGRAPHY. Because the size, shape, and structure of the kidneys are well visualized, ultrasound is a good screening examination to evaluate the size of the kidneys and to detect obstruction (blockage of the urine flow), cysts, and cancers. Further testing is usually not required after a normal ultrasound examination unless symptoms dictate continued investigation. In many situations, a CT scan may be necessary to evaluate suspicious masses that could be cancerous. The kidney ultrasound is painless, and the only sensation the patient will feel is the pressure of the transducer passing over the skin.

LIVER ULTRASONOGRAPHY. Since the advent of modern CT scan examinations, liver ultrasonography is no longer performed as often as in the past. However, it is still extensively used as a screening test to detect abnormalities. It is also performed to supplement information where results of a CT scan are equivocal. This test also has the advantage of not requiring preparation or the use of a contrast agent. It also takes less time and is less expensive than a CT scan, enhancing its value as a screening tool.

One of the prime reasons for performing ultrasonography of the liver is to detect metastatic disease, most commonly metastatic cancers of the lung, breast, and colon. The normal liver echoes can often be clearly distinguished from the abnormal echoes of cancer. Benign (nonmalignant) conditions such as cysts may be more clearly diagnosed with ultrasound than with CT scans. For this reason, an ultrasound examination may clarify equivocal CT scan findings.

Ultrasonography of the liver is frequently used to evaluate the size of the bile ducts, those tubes which lead from the liver and the gallbladder into the small intestine (duodenum). Bile-duct enlargement (dilatation) may point to such diverse diseases as stones in the bile ducts and cancer of the pancreas. The sonogram will reveal pressure on the major bile ducts causing back-up of bile and thus distension of the bile ducts.

Patients lie on their back while this painless procedure is performed. The only sensation is that of the transducer passing over the skin. The test takes about 15 minutes.

PANCREATIC ULTRASONOGRAPHY. The pancreas manufactures digestive juices, and part of the organ is adjacent to the intestine, near the point of entry of the major bile duct (common bile duct). When tumors arise in this location they may cause blockage of the bile ducts. Since jaundice (yellowing of the skin) may occur as a result of bile-duct obstruction, the pancreatic scan is often performed in conjunction with a liver ultrasound scan in order to evaluate the entire bile-duct system. Infections of the pancreas (pancreatitis) may also be clearly visualized with ultrasound.

Patients lie on their back while this painless procedure is performed. The only sensation is that of the transducer passing over the skin. The test takes about 15 minutes.

Bowel gas will interfere with the transmission of sound waves to the pancreas. For this reason, CT scans of the pancreas often supplement the pancreatic ultrasound test where findings remain equivocal.

Computed Axial Tomography Scanning
(CT Scan or CAT Scan)

Computed axial tomography—or as it is more commonly known, CT scanning—allows for the precise visualization of many abnormalities in the body. The development of the CT scan represented a major step in technology, allowing for the accurate display of disease processes and organ anatomy.

The CT scan images are created by the interaction of x-rays with body tissues. Specialized detectors installed in a doughnut-shaped machine surround the part of the body to be examined. When focused x-rays pass through the body, the density differences in the various tissues (such as bone, lung, or muscle) are perceived by the detectors, and the signals are analyzed by the computer. As the body passes through the detector site, a series of images are displayed in the form of "slices," also called tomographic sections. These pictures are most commonly obtained perpendicular to the long axis of the body (axial plane). The examination table moves slowly into the detection "doughnut" so as to obtain the picture slices.

The CT scan is a painless test, during which the patient lies on a comfortable examination couch. Many CT scans must be performed with the use of intravenous contrast agents in order to highlight certain abnormalities. When the brain or the spine is examined, an intravenous contrast agent may be required, depending on the clinical picture. Contrast agents are always injected for CT examinations of the chest unless the patients has a significant history of allergies.

For abdominal and pelvic CT scans, the patient drinks approximately one quart of oral contrast agent in order to fill the intestinal tract. To further improve accuracy, an intravenous contrast agent is injected at the time of the examination.

Side effects are related to the contrast agents, not the scanning itself. Intravenous injections may cause mild flushing and a sensation of being hot. A mild allergic reaction to the agent may cause itching; a severe reaction is rare, but is considered a medical emergency and is treated immediately.

The oral contrast agent often causes bloating and diarrhea. If a patient is very ill, this part of the examination is omitted. Unfortunately, this reduces the diagnostic accuracy of the test.

CT scan examination times average between 30 minutes and an hour. The examination room is kept cool in order for the computer to operate efficiently.

The images are displayed on a video screen, which is monitored by the technician. After the appropriate area is examined, and the study completed, the pictures are then photographed on x-ray film and analyzed by a radiologist.

The following types of CT scans are listed alphabetically.

ABDOMEN AND PELVIS. CT scans of the abdomen clearly visualize the internal organs and their relationship to one another. The stomach and other parts of the intestinal tract (including the esophagus, located in the chest) are imaged by administering a contrast agent taken orally. This fills the gastrointestinal tract to prevent these structures from being confused with abnormal masses. Although inconvenient, it is necessary for patients to drink large amounts of the contrast agent. Infections and cancers in the abdominal and pelvic regions are often clearly visualized, and frequently no additional imaging tests are needed.

Most disease states will be more cost-effectively examined by using CT scanning rather than other tests because the CT scan often results in a specific diagnosis. Ultrasound remains preferable to CT scanning for gynecological conditions because it does not involve radiation. The CT scan's advantage over other tests, including ultrasound, lies in its superior display of organ relationships to one another, particularly in evaluating the location and extent of cancers. With the exception of MRI scanning of the brain, neck, and spine and nuclear scanning of the skeleton, CT scanning is often the most cost-effective and best test for detecting and evaluating cancers of the chest, abdomen, and pelvis.

Infections in general are best detected if they form abscesses. These appear as soft-tissue masses on the CT scan, but they must be differentiated from the similar densities of adjacent bowel loops. The same holds true for cancer masses. Abscesses and cancer masses usually resemble one another on CT scans. For this reason the patient's history and physical examination are of great value in establishing a correct diagnosis.

Cancers affecting the liver, kidneys, pancreas, lymph nodes, and bile ducts are generally well demonstrated on CT scans. This is often the only type of imaging that detects these diseases.

In the pelvis, the CT scan is primarily used to diagnose cancer and its local extensions. It is also done to further evaluate an equivocal gynecologic finding first detected on an ultrasound.

CT scan is often used when lymph-node enlargement is suspected or to evaluate the result of lymph-node treatment. A lymphangiogram may still be performed occasionally, especially in the evaluation of suspected lymph-node abnormalities in Hodgkin's disease. However, it has lost some of its importance since the advent of CT scanning.

CENTRAL NERVOUS SYSTEM (BRAIN AND SPINE). MRI scans have largely replaced CT scans as the best test for neurologic (brain and spine) abnormalities. Cancers, strokes, and herniated discs are best detected with MRI. However, when this technology is not available, or to minimize cost, the CT scan is a very effective alternative.

Neurological (brain and spine) abnormalities such as cancers, strokes, and herniated discs are often clearly depicted on a CT scan. The size, location, and extent of the disease seen allows for precise medical and surgical treatment. The CT scan of neurological conditions has largely replaced many x-ray tests previously performed, some of which were very painful and dangerous.

The CT scan frequently detects neurological disease without specifically indicating its cause. In such cases, a list of possible conditions, called a differential diagnosis, may be offered. By following the *evolution* of the abnormality, the specific diagnosis becomes apparent. As a result, patients who have undergone brain CT scans may often find that follow-up scans are performed over a period of time. On occasion, patients with symptoms of early disease may have a negative (normal) scan that turns positive (abnormal) on follow-up examination as the disease progresses. A biopsy may be performed when the diagnosis remains doubtful.

CT scans of the spine have reduced the need for myelograms. Sometimes both tests may be necessary since the combination of the myelogram and CT scan may lead to greater diagnostic precision. Many patients who are thought to have a herniated disc have symptoms secondary to arthritis of the spine. Here the CT scan clearly differentiates between the two conditions and often prevents the necessity of a diagnostic myelogram.

Injuries to the brain and to a lesser extent the spinal cord are well diagnosed with a CT scan. For example, even in the absence of fractures, the skull may sustain severe injury. Thus, a negative skull x-ray does not preclude an extensive CT scan work-up of the brain. Collections of blood trapped between the skull and the brain (subdural and epidural hematomas), as well as bleeding into the brain substance, may be rapidly diagnosed using this technique, and life-saving procedures instituted. The base of the skull is more easily examined by CT scan than by conventional x-rays.

Spinal injuries are well imaged with CT scanning. This test is usually ordered for complicated spinal fractures that cannot be fully revealed through conventional x-rays. However, for most vertebral injuries conventional x-rays are sufficient. The soft tissues of the spine—that is, the spinal cord and nerve roots and their coverings—can also be imaged with the CT scan.

CT scanning can effectively image infections of the brain and spine. However, MRI scanning and biopsies may also be necessary in order to distinguish between infections and cancer. CT scans of the brain are commonly performed to detect and evaluate strokes.

The CT scan is a good initial test to evaluate a suspected brain cancer, either originating there or spreading from a distant site. MRI scanning may then be used to further clarify the extent and nature of the cancer. In most situations, however, the CT scan is an excellent test to diagnose cancer and to evaluate the results of radiation treatment.

CHEST. Although chest x-rays are valuable, when more information is necessary to confirm a diagnosis or to evaluate lymph nodes, CT scans are of inestimable value. The CT scan is particularly useful in evaluating the lymph nodes of the mediastinum (central chest tissues). Often, pneumonias mask underlying cancers, and the CT scan greatly helps in differentiating one from the other. Furthermore, this test is used to plan biopsy procedures of the mediastinal lymph nodes or lung masses as well as surgery.

Precise evaluation of the results of treatment for lung cancer can also be monitored by CT scanning, because ordinary chest x-rays are often not accurate and sensitive enough to perform this function.

Ordinary pneumonias and chronic lung diseases do not usually require the frequent use of CT scanning. Here, chest x-rays often will suffice.

CT scanning for trauma to the chest is often life-saving, because the extent of injury to the lungs, bronchial tubes, and major blood vessels can be rapidly evaluated.

HEAD AND NECK. In the evaluation of head and neck diseases, particularly those due to injury and tumor, the CT scan is usually far superior to all conventional x-ray techniques. Surgeons preparing to correct injuries to the facial bones, for example, are able to visualize the abnormalities preoperatively.

Cancer surgeons may use the CT scan to evaluate the extent of disease prior to surgery, and radiation therapists plan patients' treatment using the results of the scan. Radiation therapists also use the scans after surgery to determine the location of residual cancer. MRI scanning (see below) may eventually be the test of choice for head and neck evaluation because it more accurately images the soft tissues in the neck.

Magnetic Resonance Imaging (MRI Scanning)

Magnetic resonance imaging is one of the new high-tech fields of diagnostic radiology. It is unique because it provides precise and detailed anatomic information without exposing the patient to x-rays. To date, no biological ill effects resulting from MRI have been discovered, and many modern medical facilities now own this equipment. MRI scans are very expensive, so if physicians believe that a CT scan will provide sufficient information in a particular situation, they tend to use it instead.

Cancers, whether they originate in the brain or have spread there from distant organs, are particularly well visualized. The brain is imaged almost as it appears to the surgeon. The images are processed as "slices" of brain on x-ray film. These slices can be obtained in many different views, referred to as projections.

Although the MRI is very sensitive, it is not very specific in differentiating between cancer and infections of the brain. Therefore, the patient's history and physical findings are important in establishing a definite diagnosis. On occasion, a biopsy may be necessary to clear up any doubts.

Although MRI technology is extremely complicated, the general principle on which it is based can be simply stated. Atoms (specifically their nuclei) in the body can be made to act like bar magnets with north and south poles. This occurs when the magnetic field of the MRI machine is applied to the body. The nuclei of the hydrogen atoms in the body line up in relation to the magnetic field applied. When radio waves are transmitted into the patient, these atoms, acting as tiny magnets, tilt on their axes, resulting in some absorption of the radio waves. Hence, the term *resonance*. When the radio signal is shut off, the atoms, again acting as little magnets, return to their original state and send back the signal they absorbed. This rebroadcast is detected by an antenna, and the signal is processed by computer into an image. The magnetic field of the machine is very powerful, thousands of times greater than that of the Earth's magnetic field.

The images produced result in tissue slices, similar to the CT scan. However, MRI images are more detailed, and the test is more versatile than the CT scan in that images may be obtained in many more geometric planes. The most common planes used are the axial (perpendicular to the long axis of the body, as in slicing a loaf of bread) and the sagittal (parallel to the long axis of the body, as in slicing carrot sticks).

The following types of MRI scans are listed alphabetically.

ABDOMEN AND PELVIS. MRI and CT scans are approximately equal in accuracy for evaluating conditions of the abdomen and pelvis. As a rule, CT scans are performed because they are less expensive. Eventually, however, MRI may become the ideal test for the staging of cancer.

MRI technology is currently unable to detect small calcifications seen in kidney stones, gallstones, and certain tumors. The image is also affected by normal biological motion such as intestinal activity and breathing. As a result, the ability of MRI to evaluate the gastrointestinal tract and small masses in the lung is somewhat reduced.

BRAIN AND SPINE. For diseases of the brain and spine, the MRI scan is superior to the CT scan especially for strokes, most brain tumors, and diseases such as multiple sclerosis. The MRI scan is usually superior for diagnosis of conditions of the spine since it can image the entire spinal cord in its long axis (it looks like a tube). Its coverings and surrounding fluid (cerebrospinal fluid) are also well imaged. Thus, cancers originating in or spreading to the spine, and their compressive effects, are especially well demonstrated. This has decreased the need for CT scans and myelograms.

Recently, special contrast agents have been designed to enhance MRI images. These are used in special situations to enhance the appearance of suspected abnormalities in the brain and spine, thereby allowing a more accurate diagnosis.

CHEST. The role of MRI in detecting and evaluating lung cancer is currently being investigated. At the present time, however, the CT scan is less expensive and very accurate.

HEAD AND NECK. Because of its ability to visualize small differences in soft tissues, MRI appears to be the ideal test to evaluate cancers of head and neck. While these cancers can be examined visually, their extensions into the deeper tissues are best evaluated with MRI.

JOINTS. MRI is currently the best imaging test for the diagnosis of joint disease.

Certain conditions contraindicate the use of MRI imaging. Specifically, pacemakers may be shut down and surgical clips in the head or eyes may dislodge. In addition, patients requiring life-support systems containing metal cannot be examined because the metal is attracted to the magnet.

In the future, MRI scanning will be able to evaluate subtle chemical changes in the body's tissues. Therefore, disease processes will be identified not only by their structure, but by their chemical changes. This will lead to increased diagnostic accuracy and may decrease the need for surgical procedures such as biopsies.

&

Chapter 10

Twenty-five Frequently Asked Questions About Radiation Therapy and Cancer

1. Will I become radioactive as a result of radiation therapy?

No, this *can't* happen. The energy from the radiation is directly converted into a biochemical change. As a result, the cancer cell's ability to survive and reproduce is altered.

2. Am I dangerous to others as a result of radiation therapy?

Remember that only the cells in the irradiated part of the body are affected. The rest of the body is spared. This is *focal* treatment to a local area. It should be distinguished from *total body* irradiation, which occurs when radioactive substances are injected in the bloodstream or ingested, or when industrial accidents and other uncontrolled situations involving radiation occur. As explained above, no residual radiation energy is present in the body. Therefore, there is no way for you to pass on radiation energy to those around you.

3. Is my cancer contagious?

As far as we know, cancer is not a disease that can be transmitted to another person. This is most often a concern to people who have a cancer in a reproductive organ and wonder if a sexual partner could possibly catch the disease. It is not surprising that people wonder about this because there remain many unanswered questions about the causes of cancer. There is still a great deal of mystery about the disease, and it is perhaps the most feared disease we must contend with.

Over the years, researchers have documented cancers occurring in clusters in schools and communities. Leukemia is one example. Scientists studying the occurrence and causes of cancer have looked into many factors that could cause these clusters. To date, a direct person-to-person transmission has *never* been documented. Rather, environmental pollutants are believed to be the cause of these cancers.

Certain kinds of cancer, breast and colon in particular, are thought to be caused by genetic factors because they tend to run in families. It is essential that those in families in which these cancers appear undergo periodic cancer screening.

4. Will I die from the cancer I have?

Fifty percent of all people who have contracted their cancer in the past 10 years will *survive the disease* and live a normal life span. This statistic will undoubtedly improve as new discoveries are made relating to prevention and early detection. Treatment methods are also steadily improving, and this progress will further help increase cure rates.

Some cancers already have very high cure rates—better than 85 percent. They include breast cancer when detected in its early stages, early cancer of the vocal cords, early Hodgkin's disease, some testicular cancers, and most skin cancers.

People often view cancer as a death sentence because they have known people who died from the disease. Therefore, they think that a similar fate is inevitable. This fear of death—sometimes even an assumption of death—is one of the stages that people with cancer often go through. It is wise to admit to having the fear, talk about it, and seek help if necessary. (Cancer support groups serve an important function for many people.) Over the years, I have found that people feel better in the long run by examining their fears and dealing with the realities of cancer. By contrast, retreating into a silent denial or forcing yourself to be unrelentingly positive actually may be detrimental.

Neither you nor your physicians know when you are going to die or what the cause will be. I've observed that, ultimately, most people try to achieve the best life they can regardless of how long they will live. It seems to me that this is more important than the impersonal estimates of "time left." The statistics given, even for advanced cancers, need not prevent you from defying the odds, because cures abound.

5. My doctor told me that my cancer is advanced. Can I still achieve a good quality of life?

Most likely there are many things that can be done to make daily life as pleasant and comfortable as possible. Radiation therapy, chemotherapy, and/or surgery are often used to help control the cancer and prevent unpleasant symptoms. Medication can control the pain, diet can be modified, and emotional support systems can be developed. I have personally seen patients with very advanced cancers live relatively full lives even when the disease itself was considered hopeless. Naturally, a person's age and overall medical condition affect quality of life, but a person's spirit is important too.

6. Will I become a drug addict because I need pain medication?

There is no evidence that cancer patients become addicted to the pain-relief medication they take, at least in the way an addict is defined in today's society. That is, patients do not begin to crave the drugs for their euphoric or hallucinatory effects. Patients may, however, become physically dependent on the pain medication to do what the drug is intended to do—relieve pain. Drug dosages may be increased or decreased as warranted, and most patients stay on the same medication for long periods of time. However, medications are often reduced when cancer treatments lessen the pain.

When the disease improves, the need for medication usually decreases markedly. Either the medication is decreased in dosage, or a less potent medication is prescribed. For example, people who have been on morphine switch to aspirin or Tylenol. Patients who are cured or who even undergo long-term remissions may not need any medication. It must be emphasized that narcotic medication, when indicated and necessary for the patient's comfort, should be taken as needed for as long as it is required.

7. Will I lose my hair as a result of radiation therapy?

As a rule, radiation treatment results in scalp hair loss if the whole head is treated with doses greater than 3,000 to 4,000 units. Local scalp hair loss will occur over just the areas treated. The hair may eventually grow back, but the texture may be more fine or coarse than it was before treatment. Radiation delivered to other parts of the body may also cause local hair loss. A popular misconception is that scalp hair loss occurs regardless of the area being irradiated. However, the generalized hair loss that occurs with chemotherapy does not occur with radiation treatment.

8. What will happen to my skin during radiation therapy?

Fortunately, the technology of radiation therapy has improved in the last 40 or so years, and today's newer machines are "skin sparing." In the early days of radiation therapy (the first half of this century), patients often experienced extensive skin reactions. However, with today's technology, *mild* reddening and irritation of the skin is experienced only in the area under treatment. This irritation may particularly occur in areas where the skin rubs against skin—under the arms and the folds in the buttocks, for example. No adverse skin effects are present outside the area of treatment.

When high radiation doses are necessary, particularly in fair-skinned individuals, the skin may crack and blister. Skin creams are effective for their soothing and healing effects. These symptoms are temporary and disappear in two to four weeks after treatment is completed. The skin will darken gradually and then peel to reveal normal underlying skin, much like the effects of a sunburn. In general, darker-skinned people experience less intense skin reactions than those with very fair skin.

9. Should I take vitamin and mineral supplements during my treatment?

I recommend taking standard doses of nutritional supplements. By standard, I mean those supplements that provide the RDA (recommended daily allowance) of vitamins and minerals. The supplements are important because the diet might be limited and the ability to absorb nutrients diminished during treatment.

Some specific vitamins and minerals may be useful in higher than normal doses, but the evidence is still incomplete, and physicians differ in their attitudes about high doses of various nutrients. These supplements should be used only with medical supervision. I favor their use.

10. I have a cancer that is considered inoperable, and I will receive only radiation therapy. Does this mean there is no hope for a cure?

Most people confuse inoperable with nonoperable. *Nonoperable* means there is no need for surgery. In many cases, radiation therapy is a curative procedure without the need for surgery. In other situations, radiation therapy can result in long-term survival without the trauma of mutilating surgery. Therefore, many people should consider themselves fortunate in not undergoing surgery, that is, being "nonoperable."

Some patients are truly *inoperable*, meaning that while surgery could effect a cure for that particular cancer, in these cases, the disease is too far advanced or the person too frail for surgery to be effective. Radiation can often improve quality of life for these patients.

11. Will I lose my ability to function sexually as a result of treatment?

Some specific cancer treatments to the reproductive organs, such as radiation therapy to the prostate, may eventually lead to sexual dysfunction in a percentage of patients. Prostate surgery, for example, may result in impotence, especially when it is characterized as "radical." This applies to many pelvic cancers, specifically bladder and prostate in men. Radiation may also cause some men to become impotent. In women, external radiation therapy to the pelvis may irritate the vaginal tissues and cause enough discomfort so that intercourse is avoided temporarily. Internal radiation for cervical or uterine cancer may result in scarring of the vaginal tissues. Stretching of the tissues may be needed, and in some cases, a degree of dysfunction may be permanent.

In many cancer patients, however, sexual functioning is not directly affected. Sexual relations may continue if the patient feels well enough and depression, fatigue, and other side effects do not interfere with the desire for sexual contact.

The loss of sexual function or desire among some patients may occur as a result of feelings of shame or unattractiveness. These feelings are more common among patients who have undergone mutilating surgeries. Support groups, individual counseling, and loving relationships with sexual partners will help minimize these feelings.

12. Have I done something wrong to develop the cancer?

Some studies have demonstrated that certain personality traits or the occurrence of a catastrophic life event may predispose a person to develop cancer. However, these studies are controversial. They seem to show that a major stressful life event or a predisposition to chronic feelings of helplessness and an impaired ability to communicate can, in some people, stimulate the development of a cancer—or other major illnesses. This may be related to a generalized weakening of the immune system that makes the body more prone to disease processes of any kind, such as infections and cancers. However, there is no known psychological connection for the majority of cancer patients. Some harmful substances (such as nicotine, excess alcohol, and environmental pollutants) are known to cause cancer. I believe that it is wise for cancer patients to get on with their lives rather than wasting valuable energy on what is only speculation.

13. I am so depressed that I'm unable to cope. Is this common?

It is perfectly normal to be depressed because a diagnosis of cancer is so overwhelming. People often see it as their body's betrayal, and they have taken normal good health, up to this point, for granted. Many patients unfortunately do not exhibit or discuss this depression. However, it is important to talk about it in order to decrease anxiety. A depression may aggravate a person's condition, and to some degree, even interfere with the treatments. A positive attitude is quite helpful.

Some people attempt to deny their diagnosis. Again, it is important for patients not to internalize their fears, but rather find a way to express them. In this way, they can deal with the situation realistically. Counseling and support groups can also be very helpful. The will to live and beat the odds has been found to be an important part of stimulating the body's defenses to fight the cancer and promote healing.

14. What exactly are the lymph nodes?

Lymph nodes are small, rounded pealike structures found throughout the body. They are part of the lymph system, which contains fluid and forms a continuous channel. This channel connects to our bloodstream by an opening in a large vein in the upper chest.

The lymph nodes (often mistakenly referred to as lymph glands) and lymph channels contain a clear fluid in which white blood cells and nutrients float. The lymph nodes and channels are part of the body's defense system against disease. The nodes act as biological filters, trapping elements foreign to the body, such as infections or cancers. When a person develops tonsillitis, for example, the painful swellings felt in the neck are the lymph nodes containing the infection, which has drained through the lymphatic system from the tonsils. Similarly, cancers of various organs will drain through the lymph channels into the neighboring lymph nodes.

Once the infection or cancer is contained by the lymph nodes, there is a chance for cure if appropriate and adequate treatment stops further spread. Because the lymph-channel system connects with the bloodstream, it is easy to see why unsuccessfully treated infections and cancers can spread to distant sites in the body. Lymph nodes are part of the solution for resisting disease, but become part of the problem when overwhelmed. Thus, what starts as a local infection or cancer may in time exist elsewhere.

15. Can radiation therapy be given to an organ structure more than once?

This depends on the type of cancer and its location. Generally speaking, cancers localized to one organ, without evidence of spread beyond that organ or the adjacent lymph nodes, are given a maximum dose with the hope that the cancer will not recur in that region. The maximum dose is based upon knowledge of what dose is effective to cure or arrest the cancer as well as the tolerance of the normal tissues to the radiation. In these situations, it would be unusual for the radiation therapist to deliver additional radiation to the region.

When bones are involved, usually as a result of spread from a distant region, they may be retreated. This applies particularly to bones of the arms and legs, because those surrounding soft tissues may tolerate high doses of radiation. Each person's situation is different, and decisions are made based upon the particular clinical picture and the radiation therapist's judgment.

When cancer remains after the original dose has not been found to be sufficient, the radiation therapist will often work with a chemotherapist because drugs may eradicate disease not completely destroyed by radiation.

16. Can I shield the rest of my body during treatment to protect it from radiation?

Radiation treatments are delivered in a precisely focused way so that tissues outside those in the path of the treatment beam do not become *directly* irradiated. Once internal, some radiation may be deflected sideways, and this is known as "scatter." If scatter occurs close to the reproductive organs it can cause harm to these tissues. For example, young men undergoing treatment for cancer of the testicle may need to have a protective shield applied to the remaining testicle. The ovaries of young women may be surgically moved out of the way of the treatment beam in a procedure called oopheropexy.

17. How should I tell my family members that I have cancer?

Discussing cancer is much like discussing any serious illness. I believe that a frank and honest discussion is all that is necessary, and in most cases, family members and friends quickly rally around to provide practical and emotional support.

There are obvious exceptions to this general rule. For example, very young children may not understand that a disease can be simultaneously very serious and curable, and it may be better not to give them detailed explanations of the illness. Similarly, if a relative is older, very ill, or emotionally fragile, he or she may not be able to handle the information about a loved one. Common sense usually dictates when this is the case.

Describing a realistic but hopeful picture usually helps alleviate anxiety in patients and loved ones. Older children should not be excluded from information and discussions about treatment, side effects, and outlook. They generally handle knowledge of a loved one's illness far better than we give them credit for.

18. Should I seek the so-called alternative cures, such as those offered outside of the United States that are not approved by the Food and Drug Administration?

I advise extreme caution when embarking on a course of action that leads patients away from the conventional cancer therapies that are widely available and known to be effective in so many cases. In addition, these alternative therapies may conflict with currently accepted treatments. This is not to say that I believe that the medical establishment has all the answers. Scientific research continues in many areas of cancer treatment and the studies are carefully constructed and reported. Many of the alternative treatments claim cures, but to date they have not been scientifically validated.

19. Just how safe is radiation therapy?

It is always best not to be exposed to x-rays of any kind unless it is considered absolutely necessary. Radiologists and x-ray technicians always reduce their own occupational exposure to radiation as much as possible. However, x-ray testing is sometimes the only way to definitively diagnose a disease; radiation therapy is often the most effective treatment for cancer. In these cases, radiation can be considered life-saving.

20. What exactly are hospice centers, and how can I locate them?

By definition, hospice centers help terminally ill patients and their families. Hospice facilities sometimes house patients and family members and take physical care of the dying patient while offering emotional support. Sometimes the help is offered to patients in their own homes. Volunteers visit on a regular basis and help family caretakers and patients live as comfortably as possible during the difficult last stages of an illness. I advise contacting a local chapter of the American Cancer Society to learn more about hospice facilities in your area.

21. I am not experiencing any side effects from my radiation treatments. Does that mean they are ineffective?

There is a common belief that if a treatment isn't unpleasant it must not work—not unlike the belief that if medicine is foul-tasting it must be effective. Nothing could be further from the truth. It often surprises patients that they feel well throughout their treatment, but I always reassure them that there is no correlation between the side effects of treatment and the results.

22. How long do the beneficial effects of radiation therapy last?

Treatment is often administered because a cure is possible. If a cure is subsequently achieved, the effects of the radiation last for the duration of that person's life.

When treatment is administered for palliation—that is, to arrest the disease and alleviate symptoms rather than to eradicate the tumor—the effects may last from months to years.

Radiation therapy often shows a *lag effect*. The biological changes resulting from radiation are still active in the body long after treatments are completed. For example, patients receiving radiation to bone may experience pain relief long after the course of treatment is over. In addition, chest x-rays and CT scans often show that tumors become smaller weeks or months following treatment. This is the reason follow-up x-rays and other tests should be performed in the weeks and months after treatment has been completed.

23. Can I receive radiation treatment even though my blood count is low?

Until recently, radiation therapy had to be discontinued for weeks or months when the blood count was low. This was particularly true when the white-cell count was low, because there was no way to replenish those cells. However, patients with low red-cell counts could receive transfusions, and those with low platelet counts could receive a platelet transfusion, allowing treatment to continue.

Currently, it is possible to administer a growth factor for white blood cells. (Neupogen is an example of this new medication.) This growth factor considerably shortens the time that radiation treatments or chemotherapy must be delayed. A product called IL3 is being developed that will stimulate all the bone-marrow elements, red and white cells, and platelets. There will be new drugs, with fewer side effects, on the market in the future.

24. Where can I read about the latest medical studies of cancer treatments and cures?

The reading list in this book contains many titles that can help you understand and cope with your disease. In general, they are written for the lay audience rather than for the medical community. However, if you would like additional information, public and medical libraries have indexes that list recent scientific studies as well as reports that summarize and review the latest medical literature published about many cancers. Computer searches conducted by librarians can also provide current information about studies in progress. Your physician can also lead you to medical information if you wish to gain greater understanding of your illness.

25. Will I see my radiation therapist following the treatment course?

It is customary to see your radiation therapist at least once following completion of treatment, although facilities have varying policies about this. I see my patients three to four weeks after completion of treatment to answer remaining questions, to examine them for residual side effects, and to evaluate treatment results.

Glossary

Adjuvant chemotherapy: the use of chemotherapy in order to prevent the growth and spread of cancer that is not detected but is considered to be present.

Benign: tumor tissue that does not have the capability of spreading locally or metastasizing (the opposite of malignant).

Biopsy: a tissue sample obtained by surgery to evaluate the presence or absence of cancer. A biopsy is almost always necessary in order to plan appropriate treatment.

Bone marrow: a soft substance within the bone in which red and white blood cells and platelets are developed. Radiation therapy and chemotherapy may cause a decrease in blood cell production, one reason frequent blood counts are taken during cancer treatment.

Brachytherapy (internal radiation therapy): implanting a radioactive seed into a tumor, allowing a high dose of radiation to be delivered directly to the cancer cells, but sparing surrounding tissues from significant amounts of radiation energy.

Chemotherapy: the use of anticancer drugs to treat the disease by either killing the cells or preventing them from growing.

Contrast agent: a chemical that is used to highlight disease processes on x-ray tests, contrasting them against the background of the normal tissues.

Cure: an outcome of treatment that leaves the patient disease-free, with no likelihood of recurrence.

Diagnostic work-up: performing x-ray and other imaging tests, blood tests, and physical examinations in order to establish a diagnosis.

Differential diagnosis: a list of the most likely diagnoses for a particular set of symptoms and x-ray findings. The use of different imaging techniques often narrows the differential diagnosis to the most likely disease present.

Dose-time relationship: the relationship between the total amount of radiation delivered in the course of treatment and the period of time over which it is administered. This relationship is vital in determining the best treatment plan for a particular cancer patient. The radiation therapist is trained to judge what is the best dose to be delivered in the most advantageous time to achieve the best chance for cure or palliation. In determining the dose-time relationship, the radiation therapist also considers how well surrounding tissue will tolerate treatment.

-ectomy: the suffix to indicate removal of, as in pneumonectomy, the removal of lung; cystectomy, the removal of the bladder; mastectomy, the removal of a breast; colectomy, the removal of the intestine.

Electron beam: linear accelerator machines are capable of delivering radiation with photons (x-rays) and electrons. Each is a different type of radiation. Photons, in the energies used with linear accelerators, are very powerful, traversing great depths of tissues. Electrons traverse only for a limited distance depending on the energy used to propel them.

Fractionation: the daily dose of radiation based on the total dose divided into a particular number of daily treatments.

Gamma rays: radiation originating from unstable atomic nuclei. An example is the production of gamma rays from the isotope cobalt 60. Gamma rays have particular energies depending on the specific isotope from which they are emitted. For cobalt, this is approximately one million electron volts.

Grade: in reference to tumors, the aggressiveness of the cell type, from very low aggressiveness with slow growth pattern to very aggressive with rapid spread. Tumor grading classifications vary according to tumors.

Isotope: a radioactive substance used in diagnosis or treatment of cancer.

Linear accelerator: a radiation therapy treatment machine which, like cobalt, is used to treat cancer. This machine emits x-rays instead of gamma rays. Depending on the energy of the electron bombarding the target, varying energies of x-rays are emitted ranging from six million to 24 million electron volts in the currently used treatment machines.

Local invasion: the spread of cancer from an original site to the surrounding tissues.

Localized tumors: tumors that are contained in one particular site and have not yet spread.

Malignant cells: cancer cells that have the ability to spread locally in an uncontrolled fashion and may also spread to distant sites.

Metastasis(es): the spread of cancer from its original site to other parts of the body. Cancer cells from the primary site travel through the lymph system or the bloodstream and attach to the new site.

Palliation: treatment delivered not to cure but to arrest the disease. This may take the form of eradicating pain, bleeding, and so on.

Portal film: an x-ray film of the anatomic area that is designated to be treated with radiation.

Primary tumor: the place where the cancer originates, which is referred to regardless of the site of its eventual spread. Prostate cancer that spreads to the bone is still prostate cancer, and is not referred to as bone cancer.

Prognosis: the outcome, or outlook, for a patient's condition based on the type of tumor, the stage, the available treatments, and other factors such as the person's overall health status.

Radiation dose: the amount of x-ray or other energy absorbed by an irradiated object. This dose is recorded as Grays (Gy) or as Centigrays (CGy). Ten Gy equal 1,000 CGy. For simplification,

I refer to Centigrays as "units." When I say 1,000 units, this means 1,000 CGy.

Radiation portal, or radiation field: the area under treatment with radiation.

Radiation scatter: a change in the forward direction of particles of photons as a result of collision and interaction with tissues.

Radiation sensitivity: the response of the cell to radiation. Cancer cells that are very sensitive to radiation include seminoma and some lymphomas.

Regional involvement: the spread of cancer to areas near the original site and not to distant areas of the body.

Remission: this means that the disease is regressing and symptoms are improving.

Resistance: the opposite of radiation sensitivity (see above). Cancer cells that are particularly resistant to radiation include melanoma, a type of skin cancer.

Serial examination: obtaining x-rays sequentially to document the activity of a disease process. For example, a density in the lung field may be due to infection or tumor. Serial examinations, while the patient is taking antibiotics, will enable the physician to determine which is most likely.

Side effects: symptoms directly related to treatment, such as the side effect of nausea resulting from treatment over the stomach. Side effects are considered *acute* when they occur during treatment and subside when treatment is complete. Those symptoms that persist over a longer period of time are considered *chronic*.

Simulation: a process in which therapy is planned and defined before actual treatment begins. It can be likened to a trial run, in which specifics of treatment can be worked out prior to using the actual radiation therapy machine.

Site: the location of the tumor.

Stage: the anatomic extent of the cancer. Cancer may exist in the organ of origin, extend locally, or spread to regional tissues, then to local lymph nodes, and then to distant areas as metastases.

Systemic: having a widespread effect on the body rather than just local tissue.

Tumor: a swelling, mass, or lump that may be either benign or malignant. Samples of tumor tissue are examined or biopsied when cancer is suspected.

Type: which cell in a particular organ becomes cancerous. Thus, an organ, such as the skin, containing different types of cells will reveal different types of cancer, that is, basal cell cancer, squamous cell cancer, melanoma.

X-rays: penetrating electromagnetic radiations that are usually produced by bombarding a metallic target with fast electrons.

Symptoms and Medications

Symptoms for abdomen and pelvic treatment may duplicate each other, and medication is the same.

SKIN

For dry, itchy skin
- Nivea cream
- Talcum powder
- Cornstarch
- Alpha Keri soap
- Shower to Shower (containing cornstarch, talc, and baking soda)
- Aloe skin creams

For open, "wet" skin
- 2% gentian violet
- Hydrogen peroxide
- Vitamin A and D cream or ointment
- Cortisone ointments (hydrocortisone 1%)

TEETH

To prevent tooth decay
- Fluoride application
- Calcium phosphate solution (see your dentist)

For existing tooth decay
- Antibiotics
- Zinc peroxide applications

- Fluoride applications (see your dentist)

HEAD AND NECK

For dry mouth and thick saliva
- Humidifier
- Saltwater rinses and gargles, 1 tablespoon salt in an 8-ounce glass of warm water
- Salivart (synthetic saliva)
- Baking-soda rinses and gargles, 1 tablespoon in an 8-ounce glass of warm water
- Sour unsweetened candies, fruit pits
- Oral Balance
- Biotene dental chewing gum

For removal of dead tissue in mouth
- Hydrogen-peroxide rinses and gargles

For mouth and throat pain
- Xylocaine Viscous 2% solution
- Aspirin and glycerine

For infections
- Antibiotics, especially Nystatin for thrush

CHEST

For severe cough
- Hycodan syrup

For painful swallowing
- Avoidance of hot and cold solid foods and liquids
- Chewing foods well
- Liquid antacids

For severe pain
- Narcotics (as discussed in chapter 8)

ABDOMEN

For nausea and/or vomiting
- Compazine (prochlorperazine)
- Tigan (trimethobenzamide)
- Thorazine (chlorpromazine)

For mild heartburn
- Liquid antacids (Maalox, Gelucil)

For severe heartburn
- Tagamet (cimetidine)
- Zantac (ranitidine)

PELVIS

For diarrhea and cramps
- Lomotil (atropine and diphnoxylate)
- Imodium A-D
- Kaopectate
- Pepto-Bismol
- Paregoric
- Dietary modification (see chapter 3)

For rectal pain and burning
- Anusol-HC suppositories or cream

For severe rectal pain and burning
- Cortisone enemas

For urinary frequency (urgency and burning)
- Pyridium (phenazopyridine)
- Ditropan (oxybutynin)
- Hytrin (terazosin)

For urinary infection
- Antibiotics

For vaginal irritation
- Betadine suppositories or douche

For vaginal infection
- Antibiotics

Additional Reading

The following books will help you increase your knowledge of cancer and its treatments. Some are more technical and others provide information from the patient's perspective. All are valuable and I suggest them for both patients and family members.

The American Cancer Society Cookbook
Anne Lindsay
William Morrow and Co., 1988

Cancer Pain Management
Deborah B. McGuire, Ph.D., R.N., and
Connie H. Yabro, R.N., Editors
Grune & Stratton Inc., 1987

Choices—Realistic Alternatives in Cancer Treatment
Marion Morra and Eve Potts
Avon Books, 1987

Coping with Chemotherapy
Nancy Bruning, Ballantine, 1985

Diagnosis Cancer
Wendy Schlessel Harpham, M.D.
W. W. Norton, 1992

Diet and Cancer
William Creasey
Len & Febiger, 1985

Diet, Nutrition and Cancer
Committee on Diet, Nutrition and Cancer
Assembly of Life Sciences
National Academy Press, 1982

Everyone's Guide to Cancer Therapy *Outstanding book of its kind!
Malin Dollinger, M.D., and
Ernest H. Rosenbaum, M.D.
Somerville House Books Limited, 1991

200

The Facts About Chemotherapy
    A guide for cancer patients and their families
    Paul R. Reich, M.D., and Janice E. Metcalf, M.S.
    Consumers Union of United States, Inc., 1991

Getting Well Again
    Carl O. Simonton and
    Stephanie Matthews Simonton,
    J. P. Tarcher, 1978

Head First
    Norman Cousins
    Penguin Books, 1989

Love, Medicine and Miracles
    Bernie Siegal
    Harper Collins, 1986

Managing the Side Effects of Chemotherapy and Radiation
    Marylin J. Dodd, R.N., Ph.D.
    Prentice Hall Press, 1987

Understanding Cancer
    Remeker and Steven Leib
    Bull Publishing, 1979

OTHER RESOURCES

Many patients have mentioned that relaxation techniques are helpful when they cope with the emotional issues that are inevitable when being treated for cancer. Several patients have recommended the tapes listed below:

Healing Acceleration (Videotape - Marketed by Video Hypnosis, Valley of the Sun Video, P.O. Box 38, Malibu, CA 90265)

The Healing Waterfall (Audiotape - Marketed by Inner Directions, P.O. Box 66392, Los Angeles, CA 90066)

Release Natural Healing Forces (Audiotape - Marketed by Jonathan Parker's Gateways Institute, P.O. Box 1778, Ojai, CA 93023)

Index